TAI CHI SECRETS OF THE WŬ AND LI STYLES

Tai Chi Secrets of the Wŭ and Li Styles

Chinese Classics • Translations • Commentary

by Dr. Yang, Jwing-Ming

YMAA Publication Center
Wolfeboro, NH USA

YMAA Publication Center, Inc.
PO Box 480
Wolfeboro, NH 03894
800-669-8892 • www.ymaa.com • info@ymaa.com

ISBN 9781886969988 (print)
ISBN 9781594396687 (ebook)
ISBN 9781594394164 (hardcover)

Cover design by Katya Popova
Photos provided by the authors unless otherwise indicated.
Edited by James O'Leary

20240126

Publisher's Cataloging in Publication

(Prepared by Quality Books Inc.)

Yang, Jwing-Ming, 1946-
        Tai chi secrets of the wu and li styles : Chinese classics,
translation, commentary / by Yang, Jwing-Ming. -- 1st ed.
        p. cm.
        Includes bibliographical references and index.
        ISBN: 9781886969988 (print), ISBN: 9781594396687 (ebook),
        ISBN: 9781594394164 (hardcover)

        1. Tai chi. I. Title.
GV504.Y36 2001   613.7'148
                                        QBI01-201022

Contents

Foreword by Grandmaster Liang, Qiang-Ya v

About the Author xi

Preface xvii

Acknowledgments xxi

About Wŭ and Li Families xix

Thirteen Postures: Training Comprehension of the
  Thirteen Postures by Wŭ, Yu-Xiang 十三勢行功心解・武禹襄 1

Secret of the Four Words: Suffuse, Cover, Match, and
  Swallow by Wŭ, Yu-Xiang 四字密訣：敷、蓋、對、吞・武禹襄 13

Song of Pulling the Bow to Store the Jin
  by Wŭ, Yu-Xiang 蓄勁張弓歌・武禹襄 17

Body Maneuver by Wŭ, Yu-Xiang 身法・武禹襄 21

Thesis of Interpreting the Origin
  by Wŭ, Cheng-Qing 釋原論・武澄清 23

Thesis of the Fist by Wŭ, Cheng-Qing 拳論・武澄清 31

Song of Striking Hands by Wŭ, Cheng-Qing 打手歌・武澄清 35

A Postscript by Wŭ, Cheng-Qing 跋・武澄清 39

Thesis of Taijiquan by Wŭ, Ru-Qing 太極拳論・武汝清 43

The Secret of Withdraw and Release
  by Li, Yi-Yu 撤放密訣・李亦畬 49

Five Key Words by Li, Yi-Yu 五字訣・李亦畬 53

Important Training Keys of Stepping and Striking
  by Li, Yi-Yu 走架打手行功要言・李亦畬 61

Song of Taijiquan Applications
  by Li, Yi-Yu 太極拳體用歌・李亦畬 69

Song of Thirteen Postures by Li, Yi-Yu 十三勢歌・李亦畬 75

Secret of Eight Words by Li, Yi-Yu 八字歌・李亦畬 81

Song of Transporting and Applying Spirit and Qi
  by Li, Yi-Yu 神氣運行歌・李亦畬 91

Song of Random Circle by Li, Yi-Yu 亂環歌・李亦畬 97

The Acclamation of Taiji Sparring
  by Li, Yi-Yu 太極散手贊・李亦畬 101

References 105

Appendix: Translation and Glossary of Chinese Terms 107

Index 117

前言

－ "武術要不斷前進和創新；所有好的東西都應繼續吸取" －
梁強亞

楊俊敏博士邀我為其譯著新書《太極拳武、李氏先哲秘要》寫序，使我想起先師傅振嵩謝世之前，對我學練武術曾提出過三點要求：（一）．要繼續不間斷地練習；（二）．要不斷前進和創新；（三）．所有好的東西都應繼續吸取。一九五三年五月一日他老人家逝世後，這三點成為他對我的遺訓。在這裡，我想把它作為序言的開頭。

太極拳始見自清初傳於中國河南省溫縣陳家溝，而就在這一地一族的小範圍能傳向全國、現在傳向世界；由陳氏太極拳一個流派發展為與其特點有異的，楊氏、孫氏、武氏、吳氏、傅氏等等多種太極拳流派，這就是太極拳不斷前進和創新的見證。楊博士這次編譯的武氏太極拳創始人武禹襄及其兄弟武澄清、武汝清三人（他們三人又都是師從楊露禪－楊式太極拳的一代宗師，是太極拳創新的鼻祖）以及武氏之徒李亦畬等人的太極拳有關論著，亦正是太極拳發展的寫照。然而，各派太極拳間雖然在動作、套路、風格等方面都各成一體，但它們之間卻仍然保持著好些基本相同的技術方法和運動特點。比如在身體姿勢方面；均要求懸頂，順項、含胸拔背、沉肩垂肘、塌腕、鬆腰實腹、斂臀落胯、膝部鬆活、兩足分清虛實、全身中正安舒。在動作運動路線方面；均要求弧形運轉、節節貫串、上下相隨。達到運動圓活，銜接順暢。在動作速度和勁力上，除陳氏太極拳外，均要求以柔和緩慢為主，練習速度均勻。在整體要求方面，均要求以內在意識為主導，以意導體、以體導氣，意、氣、體三者配合協調。在技擊上，均強調在 "捨己從人" 的前題下，求得以靜制動、以柔克剛等等。

這些基本相同的技術方法和運動特點，在武、李氏先哲的著作中，運用了非常精僻的而又簡練的語言作了生動的闡述，有些還以詩詞形式來表達，使學者更具興趣和便於記憶；現在楊俊敏博士又以英文作了翻譯和由淺入深的、通俗的解釋，使外國人更易於理解這些用中國古代哲理解釋太極拳技法原理的精僻論述，這對於西方人不論學練何派太極拳，對中國武術推向西方、推向世界、對武術的發展，無疑是繼他近三十本著作之後又一種有價值的貢獻。

楊俊敏博士是我一九九六年來美之後認識的，他是一位力求進取、創新和繼續吸取新經驗的、享譽歐、美洲的中年武術家，他自一九七四年赴美至今二十多年來，甚至放棄工程師的工作、專心、積極地從事中華瑰寶－中國武術在西方的推廣工作，作為中華民族的子孫，這是難能可貴的。借助本書付梓之日，祝楊博士再次獲得成功；祝願中國武術之花開遍全世界！

梁強亞
二零零零年十一月
於美國加州屋崙市

Foreword

Grandmaster Liang, Qiang-Ya 梁強亞

Wushu must be advanced and created without stop; all
of the good contents should be absorbed continuously.

Liang, Qiang-Ya

Dr. Yang, Jwing-Ming invites me to write a foreword for his new book: *Tai Chi Secrets of Wǔ and Li Styles*. This makes me think of my master Fu, Zhen-Song's (傅振嵩) three demands about my Wushu training before he passed away: 1. Must practice continuously without stop; 2. Must advance and innovate without cease; 3. Must absorb continuously those things that are good. After my Master passed away on May 1, 1953, these three points became an important teaching guideline for me. Therefore, I would like to use them here, as the beginning of this foreword.

Taijiquan first spread out from Chen village, Wen county, Henan province, China (中國 · 河南省 · 溫縣 · 陳家溝) at the beginning of Qing dynasty (清朝). From this small territory and clan, it spread across all of China, and now to the whole world. The styles that have developed from Chen style, and which have established their own special stylistic characteristics are: Yang (楊), Sun (孫), Wǔ (武), Wu (吳), and Fu (傅) etc. This is the proof that Taijiquan has been advanced and innovated continuously. The documents Dr. Yang has translated and compiled in this book originated from the creator of Wǔ style Taijiquan, Wǔ, Yu-Xiang (武禹襄) and his two brothers, Wǔ, Cheng-Qing (武澄清) and Wǔ, Ru-Qing (武汝清)(Three of them were learning from Yang, Lu-Shan (楊露禪)—the creator of Yang style Taijiquan who was the pioneer of the Taijiquan creation), and also from their disciple, Li, Yi-Yu (李亦畬). This is again the profile of Taijiquan's development. However, although each style has its own Taijiquan postures, moving routines, and special characteristics, they still continuously carry within them the same fundamental and basic skills and special important features. For example, for the body's postures, all that is asked is:

for the head to be suspended; for the neck to be loose; to draw in the chest and arc the back; to sink the shoulders and drop the elbows; to settle the wrists; to loosen the waist with a firm abdomen (i.e., Qi is full in Lower Dan Tian); to restrain the arms and settle the Kua (胯) (i.e., inner and outside of thighs); to keep the knees loose and alive; to make the insubstantial and substantial of the two feet clearly discriminated; and to keep the entire body, from top to bottom, comfortable and harmoniously coordinated. For the moving path, in addition, all that is asked is: to maintain curving motion with turning; to keep all sections threaded together; for the top and the bottom to follow each other. Consequently, the actions are round and alive, following and connecting with each other, smoothly and in comfort. For moving with speed and the manifestation of Jin (other than in Chen style), in addition, all that is asked is: to begin with focusing on softness and slowness; and to practice with uniformity of speed. In general, this demands the use of the internal Yi (意)(i.e., wisdom mind) as the major controller, the use of Yi to control the body; the use of the body to guide the Qi; the Yi, Qi, and body coordinating with each other harmoniously. For the skills of fighting, in addition, all that is asked is: from the underlying state of "giving up the self and following the opponent," to use calmness to conquer movement, to use softness to subdue hardness, etc.

All of these fundamental and basic skills and action characteristics have been clearly and gracefully described in the documents written by Wŭ's and Li's ancestors. Some of them are even written as poems, which makes the learner more interested in the subject, and also makes them easier to remember. Now, Dr. Yang, Jwing-Ming has again translated them into English, and has included commentary as a path, leading from the shallows to the depths, so that the ancient Chinese philosophies underpinning the skills and theories referenced in these documents can be understood. For Western Taijiquan practitioners—no matter what style they learn—this work will be another valuable contribution as it will be to the popularization and development of Chinese Wushu itself.

I became acquainted with Dr. Yang, Jwing-Ming in 1996, after my arrival in the United States. He is a middle-aged Wushu expert who has put a great effort into the continuous progress, innovation, and understanding of his martial arts. He enjoys a great reputation in America and Europe. It has been more than twenty-five years since his arrival in the United States in 1974. Even after Dr. Yang obtained his doctorate degree in engineering, he went so far as to give up his engineering career to concentrate all his effort on developing Chinese Wushu in the West. For a Chinese person, this is not an easy choice. I would like to take this opportunity to congratulate Dr. Yang on his success, and also to express my wish that the flowers of Chinese Wushu might be spread around the whole world.

Liang, Qiang-Ya
November, 2000,
Oakland, CA

Note: Grandmaster Liang, Qiang-Ya was born in Canton province, China in 1931. He started his Wushu training with Grandmaster Fu, Zhen-Song (1881-1953) in 1945. He is an expert in Baguazhang and Wudang Taijiquan. Grandmaster Liang has been one of the most renowned Wushu masters in China. He immigrated to the United States in 1996, and currently resides in Oakland, CA. Grandmaster Liang is considered to be a pioneer in developing Chinese martial arts in the West during the past five years.

About the Author

Dr. Yang, Jwing-Ming, Ph.D. 楊俊敏博士

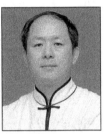

Dr. Yang, Jwing-Ming was born on August 11th, 1946, in Xinzhu Xian (新竹縣), Taiwan (台灣), Republic of China (中華民國). He started his Wushu (武術)(Gongfu or Kung Fu, 功夫) training at the age of fifteen under the Shaolin White Crane (Bai He, 少林白鶴) Master Cheng, Gin-Gsao (曾金灶)(1911-1976). Master Cheng originally learned Taizuquan (太祖拳) from his grandfather when he was a child. When Master Cheng was fifteen years old, he started learning White Crane from Master Jin, Shao-Feng (金紹峰), and followed him for twenty-three years until Master Jin's death.

In thirteen years of study (1961-1974) under Master Cheng, Dr. Yang became an expert in the White Crane Style of Chinese martial arts, which includes both the use of barehands and of various weapons such as saber, staff, spear, trident, two short rods, and many other weapons. With the same master he also studied White Crane Qigong (氣功), Qin Na (or Chin Na, 擒拿), Tui Na (推拿) and Dian Xue massages (點穴按摩), and herbal treatment.

At the age of sixteen, Dr. Yang began the study of Yang Style Taijiquan (楊氏太極拳) under Master Kao, Tao (高濤). After learning from Master Kao, Dr. Yang continued his study and research of Taijiquan with several masters and senior practitioners such as Master Li, Mao-Ching (李茂清) and Mr. Wilson Chen (陳威伸) in Taipei (台北). Master Li learned his Taijiquan from the well-known Master Han, Ching-Tang (韓慶堂), and Mr. Chen learned his Taijiquan from Master Zhang, Xiang-San (張祥三). Dr. Yang has mastered the Taiji barehand sequence, pushing hands, the two-man fighting sequence, Taiji sword, Taiji saber, and Taiji Qigong.

When Dr. Yang was eighteen years old he entered Tamkang College (淡江學院) in Taipei Xian to study Physics. In college he began the study of traditional Shaolin Long Fist (Changquan or Chang Chuan, 少林長拳) with Master Li, Mao-Ching at the Tamkang College

Guoshu Club (淡江國術社)(1964-1968), and eventually became an assistant instructor under Master Li. In 1971 he completed his M.S. degree in Physics at the National Taiwan University (台灣大學), and then served in the Chinese Air Force from 1971 to 1972. In the service, Dr. Yang taught Physics at the Junior Academy of the Chinese Air Force (空軍幼校) while also teaching Wushu. After being honorably discharged in 1972, he returned to Tamkang College to teach Physics and resumed study under Master Li, Mao-Ching. From Master Li, Dr. Yang learned Northern Style Wushu, which includes both barehand (especially kicking) techniques and numerous weapons.

In 1974, Dr. Yang came to the United States to study Mechanical Engineering at Purdue University. At the request of a few students, Dr. Yang began to teach Gongfu (Kung Fu), which resulted in the foundation of the Purdue University Chinese Kung Fu Research Club in the spring of 1975. While at Purdue, Dr. Yang also taught college-credited courses in Taijiquan. In May of 1978 he was awarded a Ph.D. in Mechanical Engineering by Purdue.

In 1980, Dr. Yang moved to Houston to work for Texas Instruments. While in Houston he founded Yang's Shaolin Kung Fu Academy, which was eventually taken over by his disciple Mr. Jeffery Bolt after moving to Boston in 1982. Dr. Yang founded Yang's Martial Arts Academy (YMAA) in Boston on October 1, 1982.

In January of 1984 he gave up his engineering career to devote more time to research, writing, and teaching. In March of 1986 he purchased property in the Jamaica Plain area of Boston to be used as the headquarters of the new organization, Yang's Martial Arts Association. The organization has continued to expand, and, as of July 1st 1989, YMAA has become just one division of Yang's Oriental Arts Association, Inc. (YOAA, Inc.).

In summary, Dr. Yang has been involved in Chinese Wushu since 1961. During this time, he has spent thirteen years learning Shaolin White Crane (Bai He), Shaolin Long Fist (Changquan), and Taijiquan. Dr. Yang has more than thirty-two years of instructional experience: seven years in Taiwan, five years at Purdue University, two years in Houston, Texas, and eighteen years in Boston, Massachusetts.

In addition, Dr. Yang has also been invited to offer seminars around the world to share his knowledge of Chinese martial arts and Qigong. The countries he has visited include Argentina, Austria, Barbados, Belgium, Bermuda, Botswana, Canada, Chile, England, France, Germany, Holland, Hungary, Ireland, Italy, Latvia, Mexico, Poland, Portugal, Saudi Arabia, Spain, South Africa, Switzerland, and Venezuela.

Since 1986, YMAA has become an international organization, which currently includes 51 schools located in Argentina, Belgium, Canada, Chile, England, France, Holland, Hungary, Ireland, Italy, Poland, Portugal, South Africa, Spain, Venezuela and the United States. Many of Dr. Yang's books and videotapes have been translated into languages such as French, Italian, Spanish, Polish, Czech, Bulgarian, Russian, Hungarian, and Iranian.

Dr. Yang has published twenty-seven other volumes on the martial arts and Qigong:

1. *Shaolin Chin Na;* Unique Publications, Inc., 1980.
2. *Shaolin Long Fist Kung Fu;* Unique Publications, Inc., 1981.
3. *Yang Style Tai Chi Chuan;* Unique Publications, Inc., 1981.
4. *Introduction to Ancient Chinese Weapons;* Unique Publications, Inc., 1985.
5. *Qigong for Health and Martial Arts;* YMAA Publication Center, 1985.
6. *Northern Shaolin Sword;* YMAA Publication Center, 1985.
7. *Tai Chi Theory and Martial Power;* YMAA Publication Center, 1986.
8. *Tai Chi Chuan Martial Applications;* YMAA Publication Center, 1986.
9. *Analysis of Shaolin Chin Na;* YMAA Publication Center, 1987.
10. *Eight Simple Qigong Exercises for Health;* YMAA Publication Center, 1988.
11. *The Root of Chinese Qigong—The Secrets of Qigong Training;* YMAA Publication Center, 1989.

12. *Muscle/Tendon Changing and Marrow/Brain Washing Chi Kung—The Secret of Youth;* YMAA Publication Center, 1989.

13. *Hsing Yi Chuan—Theory and Applications;* YMAA Publication Center, 1990.

14. *The Essence of Taiji Qigong—Health and Martial Arts;* YMAA Publication Center, 1990.

15. *Qigong for Arthritis;* YMAA Publication Center, 1991.

16. *Chinese Qigong Massage—General Massage;* YMAA Publication Center, 1992.

17. *How to Defend Yourself;* YMAA Publication Center, 1992.

18. *Baguazhang—Emei Baguazhang;* YMAA Publication Center, 1994.

19. *Comprehensive Applications of Shaolin Chin Na— The Practical Defense of Chinese Seizing Arts;* YMAA Publication Center, 1995.

20. *Taiji Chin Na—The Seizing Art of Taijiquan;* YMAA Publication Center, 1995.

21. *The Essence of Shaolin White Crane;* YMAA Publication Center, 1996.

22. *Back Pain—Chinese Qigong for Healing and Prevention;* YMAA Publication Center, 1997.

23. *Ancient Chinese Weapons;* YMAA Publication Center, 1999.

24. *Taijiquan—Classical Yang Style;* YMAA Publication Center, 1999.

25. *Tai Chi Secrets of Ancient Masters;* YMAA Publication Center, 1999.

26. *Taiji Sword—Classical Yang Style;* YMAA Publication Center, 1999.

27. *Tai Chi Secrets of Wǔ & Li Styles;* YMAA Publication Center, 2001.

Dr. Yang has also published the following videotapes:

1. *Yang Style Tai Chi Chuan and Its Applications;* YMAA Publication Center, 1984.
2. *Shaolin Long Fist Kung Fu—Lien Bu Chuan and Its Applications;* YMAA Publication Center, 1985.
3. *Shaolin Long Fist Kung Fu—Gung Li Chuan and Its Applications;* YMAA Publication Center, 1986.
4. *Shaolin Chin Na;* YMAA Publication Center, 1987.
5. *Wai Dan Chi Kung — The Eight Pieces of Brocade;* YMAA Publication Center, 1987.
6. *The Essence of Tai Chi Chi Kung;* YMAA Publication Center, 1990.
7. *Qigong for Arthritis;* YMAA Publication Center, 1991.
8. *Qigong Massage—Self Massage;* YMAA Publication Center, 1992.
9. *Qigong Massage—With a Partner;* YMAA Publication Center, 1992.
10. *Defend Yourself 1—Unarmed Attack;* YMAA Publication Center, 1992.
11. *Defend Yourself 2—Knife Attack;* YMAA Publication Center, 1992.
12. *Comprehensive Applications of Shaolin Chin Na 1;* YMAA Publication Center, 1995.
13. *Comprehensive Applications of Shaolin Chin Na 2;* YMAA Publication Center, 1995.
14. *Shaolin Long Fist Kung Fu—Yi Lu Mai Fu & Er Lu Mai Fu;* YMAA Publication Center, 1995.
15. *Shaolin Long Fist Kung Fu—Shi Zi Tang;* YMAA Publication Center, 1995.
16. *Taiji Chin Na;* YMAA Publication Center, 1995.
17. *Emei Baguazhang—1; Basic Training, Qigong, Eight Palms, and Applications;* YMAA Publication Center, 1995.
18. *Emei Baguazhang—2; Swimming Body Baguazhang and Its Applications;* YMAA Publication Center, 1995.

19. *Emei Baguazhang—3; Bagua Deer Hook Sword and Its Applications;* YMAA Publication Center, 1995.

20. *Xingyiquan—12 Animal Patterns and Their Applications;* YMAA Publication Center, 1995.

21. *24 and 48 Simplified Taijiquan;* YMAA Publication Center, 1995.

22. *White Crane Hard Qigong;* YMAA Publication Center, 1997.

23. *White Crane Soft Qigong;* YMAA Publication Center, 1997.

24. *Xiao Hu Yan—Intermediate Level Long Fist Sequence;* YMAA Publication Center, 1997.

25. *Back Pain—Chinese Qigong for Healing and Prevention;* YMAA Publication Center, 1997.

26. *Scientific Foundation of Chinese Qigong;* YMAA Publication Center, 1997.

27. *Taijiquan—Classical Yang Style;* YMAA Publication Center, 1999.

28. *Taiji Sword—Classical Yang Style;* YMAA Publication Center, 1999.

29. *Chin Na in Depth—Course One;* YMAA Publication Center, 2000.

30. *Chin Na in Depth—Course Two;* YMAA Publication Center, 2000.

31. *San Cai Jian & Its Applications;* YMAA Publication Center, 2000.

32. *Kun Wu Jian & Its Applications;* YMAA Publication Center, 2000.

33. *Qi Men Jian & Its Applications;* YMAA Publication Center, 2000.

34. *Chin Na in Depth—Course Three;* YMAA Publication Center, 2001.

35. *Chin Na in Depth—Course Four;* YMAA Publication Center, 2001.

36. Twelve Routines of Tan Tui; YMAA Publication Center, 2001.

Preface

In the last seven centuries, many songs and poems have been composed about Taijiquan. These have played a major role in preserving the knowledge and wisdom of the masters, although in many cases the identity of the authors and the dates of origin have been lost. Since many Chinese people of previous centuries were illiterate, many of the key points of the art were put into poems and songs, which are easier to remember than prose, and passed down orally from teacher to student. Treatises, which usually are more profound than the poems and songs, were also passed down. These documents were regarded as secret, and it was only in the twentieth century that they were revealed to the general public.

Almost all of the documents currently available can be categorized into five groups. The first group is the most general; it includes the most ancient documents, written either by known or unknown authors, and also those authors who do not belong to a specific style. The second to the fifth groups are comprised of those poems, songs, or treatises passed down by ancestors of Wǔ (武) and Li (李), Wu (吳), Yang (楊), and Chen (陳) families. This book will introduce the second group with eighteen poems, songs, and treatises. Many of these are the most popular of their kind, and are the most accurate in presenting the art of Taijiquan. In the near future, the other groups of documents will be translated and presented.

It should come as no surprise to the reader that it is very difficult to translate ancient Chinese writings into modern English. Because of the cultural differences, many expressions simply do not make any sense, if translated literally. Often, knowledge of the historical context is necessary. Furthermore, since every sound has several possible meanings, anybody who has ever tried to reduce these poems to writing has had to choose from among these different meanings. Over the course of several generations, this has led to variation among the poems. The same problem occurs when the poems are read. Many Chinese characters have several possible meanings, so reading involves interpretation of the text, even for the Chinese. Also, the meaning of many words has changed over the course of time. When you add to this the grammatical differences (generally, no tenses, no articles, no distinction between singular and plural, and no differentiation between parts of speech) it becomes almost impossible to provide a literal translation from Chinese to English.

With these difficulties in mind, I have attempted to convey as much of the original meaning of the Chinese as possible, based on my own thirty-eight years of Taiji experience and understanding. Although it is impossible to totally translate the original meaning, I feel that I have managed to express the majority of the important points. The translation has been made as close to the original Chinese as possible, including such things as double negatives and, sometimes, idiosyncratic sentence structure. Words that are understood but not actually written in the Chinese text have been included in parentheses. Also, some Chinese words are followed by the English in parentheses, e.g., Shen (Spirit) and some English words are followed by original Chinese, e.g., Essence (Jing). To further assist the reader, I have included commentary with each poem, song, and treatise. For your further reference, the original Chinese of each document is included. A glossary of Chinese terms is included in Appendix A for your convenience.

About Wǔ and Li Families[1,2]

The first thing you should know is not to confuse Wu style (吳氏) and Wǔ style (武氏) Taijiquan. Though the English spellings are the same, the Chinese is very different. The Wu style (吳氏) was created by Wu, Quan-You (吳全佑)(1834-1902 A.D.). The Wǔ style (武氏) was created by Wǔ, Yu-Xiang (1812-1880 A.D.)(武禹襄). The following theses and poems were originated from Wǔ style (武氏) and his student Li, Yi-Yu (1832-1892 A.D.)(李亦畬).

Wǔ, Yu-Xiang, also named: He-Qing (河清), was born in Yong Nian County, Hebei province (河北省永年). His father and grandfather were all good at scholarship and martial arts, therefore, he had been heavily influenced by them and favored martial arts himself. Around 1850 A.D. Wǔ, Yu-Xiang learned Chen style old posture Taijiquan (陳氏老架太極拳) from Yang, Lu-Shan (楊露禪). Yang, Lu-Shan was the creator of Yang style Taijiquan. In 1852, when he passed Hui-Qing County, Zhao-Bao Town, Henan (河南懷慶府趙堡鎮), he also learned Chen style new posture (陳氏新架太極拳) from Chen, Qing-Ping (陳青萍).

It is said, in 1852, his brother Wǔ, Cheng-Qing (武澄清) obtained the secret classic, *The Manual of Taijiquan* (太極拳譜) written by Wang, Zong-Yue (王宗岳). He loved it so much, he studied and pondered continuously, wrote down every comprehension, and hung them on the walls. This had brought his understanding of Taijiquan to a profound level. He wrote a few theses which include: Thirteen Postures: Comprehending External and Internal Training (十三勢行功心解), Secret of Four Words (四字不傳密訣), Important Keys of Striking Hands (打手要言), and The Ten Important Body Maneuvers (身法十要). In his life, he taught only a few students. The best student he taught was his nephew, Li, Jing-Lun (李經綸)(also named Li, Yi-Yu, 李亦畬).

Not only had Wǔ, Yu-Xiang reached a profound level of Taijiquan, his oldest brother, Wǔ, Cheng-Qing (武澄清) and second oldest brother, Wǔ, Ru-Qing (武汝清) were also known Taijiquan masters at that time.[13] Some of Wǔ, Cheng-Qing writings are: Thesis of Interpreting the Origin (釋原論), Thesis of the Fist (拳論), Song of Striking Hands

(打手歌), A Postscript (跋). Wŭ, Ru-Qing's writing includes: *Thesis of Taijiquan* (太極拳論).

Li, Yi-Yu (李亦畬), also named Li, Jing-Lun (李經綸) (1832-1892 A.D.) was born in Yong Nian County, Hebei province (河北省永年). When he was 22 years old, he started to learn Taijiquan from his uncle, Wŭ, Yu-Xiang, and became the best student who comprehended the deep theory of Taijiquan. His writings include: The Secret of Withdraw and Release (撤放密訣), Five Key Words (五字訣), Important Keys of Stepping and Striking (走架行功要言), Song of Taijiquan Applications (太極拳體用歌), Song of Thirteen Postures (十三勢歌), Secret of Eight Words (八字歌), Song of Transporting and Applying Spirit and Qi (神氣運行歌), Song of Random Circle (亂環歌), The Acclamation of Taiji Sparring (太極散手贊), The Small Foreword of Taijiquan (太極拳小序). From this, you can see that Li style originated from Wŭ's style.

Thanks to Erik Elsemans for proofing the manuscript and contributing many valuable suggestions. Thanks also to the editor, James O'Leary.

Thirteen Postures: Training Comprehension of the Thirteen Postures[1,2,6-8]

Wǔ, Yu-Xiang

十
三
勢
行
功
心
解

武
禹
襄

Use the Xin (heart, mind) to transport the Qi, (the mind) must be sunk (steady) and calm, then (the Qi) can condense (deep) into the bones. Circulate the Qi throughout the body, (Qi) must be smooth and fluid, then it can easily follow the mind.

以心行氣，務令沈著，乃能收斂入骨。以氣運身，
務令順隨，乃能便利從心。

When the Xin (心)(heart, mind) wants to do something, the Yi (will, 意) mobilizes the Qi (氣). In Taijiquan practice, where the mind goes, the Qi goes. When transporting (guiding) the Qi through your body, the mind must be clear, steady, and calm. Then, the Qi can circulate deep into the bones.

The power used in Taijiquan applications is called Jin (勁). If the Jin is united with and supported by Qi, it can reach its highest level. However, if it is not coordinated with and supported by Qi, the Jin will come only from the posture's skeletal and muscular stance. The Jin that is supported by Qi has many variations. It can range from Jins which function on the skin such as Listening Jin (Ting Jin, 聽勁), Understanding Jin (Dong Jin, 懂勁), and Adhering Jin (Zhan Jin, 粘勁), to Jins which come from deep within the bones, where offensive Jins such as Wardoff Jin (Peng Jin, 掤勁) are generated. If the Qi cannot reach deep into the bones, the Jin will lose its internal Qi support and become merely external dynamic force.

When Qi circulates throughout the body in Taiji practice and meditation, it must not be stagnant or discontinuous. In time the Qi will flow smoothly and quickly to the place where it is required. In the beginning, this will be difficult. After years of correct practice, Qi can be used to support Jin whenever the mind wishes.

(If) the Spirit of Vitality (Jing-Shen) can be raised, then (there is) no delay or heaviness (clumsiness). That means the head is suspended. Yi (Mind) and Qi must exchange skillfully, then you have gained the marvelous trick of roundness and aliveness. This means the substantial and the insubstantial can vary and exchange.

精神能提得起，則無遲重之虞。所謂頂頭懸也。意
氣須換得靈，乃有圓活之妙。所謂變轉虛實也。

The Taijiquan Classic by Wang, Zong-Yue (王宗岳) states "An insubstantial energy leads the head upward." If you cultivate this feeling, which is like having the head and body suspended by a thread, and balance this with the Qi sunk deeply into the Lower Dan Tian (Xia Dan Tian, 下丹田), then the postures will be erect and straight, and the Spirit of Vitality (Jing-Shen)(精神) will be able to rise to the top of the head. The Spirit of Vitality is the basic Spiritual vital energy of your body. When you lift this energy to the top of your head, your postures will be firmly rooted and you will be alert and responsive; therefore there will be no delay or clumsiness. When the mind and Qi are coordinated, then your skill and techniques can be round, smooth, and alive. Therefore, you can easily move yourself to exchange substantial and insubstantial in response to your opponent's actions.

When emitting Jin, be calm and relaxed, concentrated in one direction. When standing, the body must be centered, calm and comfortable, so you can handle the eight directions.

發勁須沈著鬆淨，專注一方。立身須中正安舒支撐
八面。

When using Jin to attack, your mind must be calm and your body relaxed, i.e., your movement and circulation must be unhindered and unrestrained. Taiji Jin acts like a soft whip. If you are tensed, the Jin manifested will be stagnant and not penetrating. Your attention and your energy must be concentrated and focused in the target. Taijiquan specializes in attacking the cavities. If the Jin is not focused in the cavities, it will not be effective. Through attacking the cavities, the internal organs will be shocked. That is why it is said the Taiji power penetrates into the internal organs.

Your body should be erect, centered, and stable, and should not lean to any side. If you are calm and relaxed, and your postures natural and comfortable, you will be able to deal with attacks from any direction without resistance or stagnation.

Transport Qi as though through a pearl with a "nine-curved hole," not even the tiniest place won't be reached. When using Jin, (it is) just like steel refined 100 times: no solid (strong opposition) can resist destruction.

行氣如九曲珠，無微不到。運勁如百鍊鋼，無堅不摧。

When you build up your Qi and have achieved "Small Circulation" (Xiao Zhou Tian, 小周天), you must accomplish "Grand Circulation" (Da Zhou Tian, 大周天) and fill the entire body with Qi. When you use Jin, Qi must support it. Jin and Qi should not be separated. A Chinese emperor had a large pearl that he wanted to put on a string. However, the hole through the pearl was not straight, but instead had nine curves. It was impossible to push a string through it. A wise man finally tied a very fine thread to an ant, and caused the ant to walk through this nine-curved channel pulling the thread. In the same fashion, your mind must lead the Qi throughout your body from the skin to deep inside the bones until it reaches every last part. When you cultivate your Qi, you can develop an internal (Qi supported) energy called Nei Jin (內勁)(i.e., internal Jin), which is far superior to external, or purely muscular, strength. This Jin will enable you to overcome and destroy any opposition, no matter how strong or hard.

The appearance (of the attack) is like an eagle catching a rabbit, the Spirit is like a cat catching a mouse.

形如搏兔之鶻，神似捕鼠之貓。

An eagle circles high in the air, watching for prey. When it sees a rabbit it suddenly plunges down, appearing out of nowhere to snatch its prey. When a cat sees a mouse it doesn't attack at once, but instead stalks it, biding its time till the right opportunity presents itself. While poised and watching, the cat is the very model of Spirit—alert, vital, centered, and controlled.

(Be) calm like a mountain, move like a river.

靜如山岳，動如江河。

Your Spirit and posture must be calm and stable like a mountain. Any motion large or small should flow like a river—continuous and fluid.

Accumulate Jin like drawing a bow, emit Jin like (a bow) shooting an arrow.

蓄勁如張弓，發勁如放箭。

You accumulate energy by bending like a bow, and then snap straight, propelling your opponent away. Remember that you must draw the bow before you can shoot the arrow, and you must accumulate energy before you can emit it. Here "accumulate" implies two things: 1. Qi is generated and accumulated at the Lower Dan Tian and condensed in the spine for supporting the Jin. 2. Jin is stored in the most advantageous posture to either neutralize or attack.

Find the straight in the curved; accumulate, then emit.

曲中求直，蓄而後發。

Store Jin in the curves and coils of your posture, but emit Jin in a straight line. When an opponent attacks, move your body to evade him and accumulate energy, and then snap straight to attack. Similarly, you can curve the opponent's attack away from your body, and then emit force to send him off on a tangent or right angle. Your counterattack comes out of the neutralization of his attack. You accumulate energy from his pressure, then release it.

Power is emitted from the spine; steps change following the body.

力由脊發，步隨身換。

"Power" here is Nei Jin Li (內勁力). Nei Jin (內勁) means internal energy and Li (力) means muscular strength. Any movement requires Li, and this is all that most people ever use. When you train your internal energy through meditation, Qigong, and the Taijiquan form, you can develop an energy in which the muscles are supported more and more by Qi. The spine is the major path of Qi. When Qi is built up in the Lower Dan Tian it will pass through the Sea Bottom (Haidi)(海底) and tailbone (Weilu)(尾閭), follow the spine up to the shoulders, and finally move into the arms and hands for defense and offense. If you are familiar with Grand Circulation in Taijiquan, whenever you wish to enhance the Jin's manifestation, you will also open the Mingmen

(命門)(Gv-4) cavity and lead extra Qi from the Lower Dan Tian, along the spine upward to the arms. Therefore, the Lower Dan Tian is the source of Qi, but the spine is the distributor of the Qi from where it is extended to the arms. When Taijiquan is to be used for fighting, you should not only acquire Jin with strong Qi support, but also develop a fighting strategy. This is extremely important, for a good Taiji fighter uses footwork to position his body most advantageously for each technique.

To collect is to release; to release is to collect; broken, then reconnected.

收即是放，放即是收。斷而復連。

Just as you bend a bow and then release it, you accumulate energy and then emit it. When you neutralize an attack your counterattack, should follow immediately. The one leads to the other as Yin leads to Yang. Immediately after emitting Jin, the Jin is said to be "broken." But your Yi (concentration) is not broken, and its continuity restores the Jin.

Back and forth (with the opponent) must have folding and mutual entwining. Advancing and withdrawing must have rotation and variation.

往復須有摺疊，進退須有轉換。

When you are pushing hands or sparring, you are exchanging techniques back and forth. You must be flexible and adaptable, folding and bending as appropriate. When you attack with the hand and the hand is deflected, you "fold" and attack with the elbow. If the elbow is blocked, you fold again and attack with the shoulder. "Folding" can also refer to the spiraling motion of Chan Si Jin (纏絲勁)

(silk reeling energy). "Mutual entwining" refers to when your arms are wrapping around your opponent's arms, and you are twisting and twining around, trying to gain an advantage. This is like the child's game where you put your hand out, palm down, and the other person puts his hand on top of yours. You then put your other hand on top of his, he puts a hand on top of yours, and on and on.

When you advance and withdraw during attack and neutralization, you must be rotating your waist and varying your steps. You move in different directions and change your techniques in infinite variation.

(Fist) extremely soft, then extremely hard. If able to breathe (properly), then (you) can be agile and alive.

極柔軟，然後極堅剛。能呼吸，然後能靈活。

Before you can be hard, you must first cultivate softness. Only through complete relaxation can you develop your Qi and become supremely sensitive and responsive to your opponent's actions. Only by learning not to rely on external muscular strength (Li) can you develop your internal energy and achieve real strength. It is necessary to learn how to breathe properly, that is, to develop your Qi, and then coordinate your actions with your breathing and your Qi. Only then can you be truly agile, responsive, and alive.

Cultivate Qi straight (i.e., naturally), no harm; Jin can be coiled and accumulated, (and) still have surplus.

氣以直養而無害，勁以曲蓄而有餘。

If you develop your Qi naturally, there will be no danger. You must proceed slowly and patiently, step by step. Don't push too hard, or try to do advanced techniques before you have completed all the preceding steps. When you move correctly, your energy is alternately coiling up and expanding. It is possible to accumulate energy, and at the same time have enough to move around and attack.

The Xin (heart, mind) is the order, the Qi is the message flag, and the waist is the banner.

心為令，氣為旂，腰為纛。

In ancient Chinese armies, when the general sent an order to a subordinate, the messenger carried a message flag so that the subordinate commander could be sure that the order came from the general. The banner refers to the flag that this sub-unit followed into battle. In Taijiquan the mind is the leader and directs the Qi. The waist leads the whole body into action.

First look to expanding, then look to compacting, then (you) approach perfection.

先求開展，後求緊湊，可臻於縝密矣。

When you begin practicing, first make the movements and postures large and open. As you progress, the movements and postures, and the circles they contain, become smaller and smaller until eventually you function with almost no motion at all. At this time your defense will have no gaps, and your attacks will be certain. In Taijiquan society, it is known that the smaller the defense circle and the higher the posture, the higher the art and the harder it is to achieve. It is simply more difficult to defend against an opponent whose Jin has already so closely reached to your body. However, if you have reached a deep level, even if there is a small circle, you can defend yourself. The advantage of the small circle defense is that once your opponent's attacking Jin has been emitted, it will be harder for him to change his mind and change the attack into defense. Therefore, if you can use the smaller circle in Taijiquan, you have the capability to defeat your opponent.

———————

It is also said: the opponent does not move, I do not move; the opponent moves slightly, I move first. Appears relaxed, but not relaxed; seems extended, but not extended. Jin (can be) broken, mind not broken.

又曰：彼不動，己不動，彼微動，己先動。似鬆非鬆，將展未展，勁斷意不斷。

Your actions are determined entirely by what the opponent does. If he doesn't move, you don't move either. However, all of your attention is concentrated on him, so that when he begins to move you can immediately act with certain effectiveness, because you are aware of his intention. In Taiji practice, you first build up Listening and Understanding Jins. Once you have mastered them, you will be able to sense and understand your opponent's intention even if he only moves slightly. Once you sense the opponent's intention, you should seize the opportunity, and move fast and first before the opponent's Jin is emitted. If you catch him when his mind is intent upon attacking, he will not be able to easily switch to a defensive mode of thought. This is how it is possible to deflect a force of one thousand pounds with a force of four ounces. Both your Spirit and posture may look relaxed, but they are alert. Your Jin and postures look extended, but they are restrained. When you emit Jin, there is a momentary break until you recover, but the continuity of your attention is not disturbed.

———————

It is also said: first in the Xin (heart, mind), then in the body; the abdomen (is) relaxed and clear (sunken); the Qi condenses into the bones; the Spirit is comfortable and the body is calm; remember this in the heart at all times. Do remember: one part moves, every part moves; one part still, every part still.

又曰：先在心，後在身，腹鬆淨，氣斂入骨，神舒體靜，刻刻存心。切記一動無有不動，一靜無有不靜。

The mind leads the body. First you must quiet your mind, then the body can be calm. The abdomen is relaxed and sunken. The imagery of the Chinese is that of water that is clear because it is still and all the impurities have sunk to the bottom. When you do this, the Qi can circulate throughout the body and penetrate into the bones, making them strong. Condensing the Qi into the bone marrow is the key to storing the Qi.

Remember, the body always moves as a unit. Don't push with just a hand or arm, push with your entire body, mind, and Spirit. When you are still, be totally still, with no stray motions.

(The mind) leads the Qi flowing back and forth, adhering to the back, then condensing into the spine; strengthen the Spirit of Vitality (Jing-Shen) internally, and express externally peacefully and easily.

牽動往來氣貼背，而練入脊骨，內固精神，外示安逸。

As the mind leads and circulates the Qi, it accumulates in the back and penetrates into the spine. As mentioned, the spine is the distributor in the application of Qi to techniques. As you continue to practice and pay attention carefully, the Spirit of Vitality will be strengthened. Be aware of all that is around you, but keep centered on your Lower Dan Tian. When you express your will in an external motion, move efficiently and peacefully.

Step like a cat walks; applying Jin is like drawing silk from a cocoon.

邁步如貓行，運勁如抽絲。

A cat steps carefully and quietly. Touch the ground lightly with your foot before you put your weight forward. When applying Jin, your Yi and Qi should be smooth and continuous, as though you are drawing a fragile thread of silk from a cocoon.

(Throughout your) entire body, your mind is on the Spirit of Vitality (Jing-Shen), not on the Qi. (If concentrated) on the Qi, then stagnation. A person who concentrates on Qi has no Li (strength); a person who cultivates Qi (develops) pure hardness (power).

全身意在精神，不在氣。在氣則滯，有氣者無力，
養氣者純剛。

Here "Qi" refers to both breath and Qi (intrinsic energy) because breathing is used to control the circulation of Qi. In the beginning of your training you must consciously coordinate your movement, breath, and Qi. However, this coordination must become automatic so that you can concentrate on the Spirit of Vitality. The mind leads the Qi, which leads the body. However, if you have to pay attention to the Qi or breathing, that means you are still regulating your Qi or breathing. When your mind is on the Qi or breathing, then the Qi is stagnant. Therefore, the strength which is generated from the Qi manifestation will be weak and clumsy. However, if you have already cultivated the Qi to a high level, and have reached the stage of regulating without regulating, then your mind will be on the Spirit of Vitality or on the opponent. When this happens, Qi is strongly led by the mind, and, when necessary, the power manifestation can be very powerful, and as strong as steel. You should remember, cultivating the Qi is only the beginning stage of power manifestation. If your mind is still on the cultivation of Qi, that means you are still at the beginning stage of your Taijiquan.

The Qi is like a cartwheel, the waist is like an axle.

氣如車輪，腰似車軸。

When you move, your waist directs the rolling, flowing Qi. Following the waist's movement, the Qi is led by the mind to the desired area of the physical body for Jin manifestation. Where and when the mind goes, the Qi goes. But all of this is governed and directed by the waist.

Secret of the Four Words: Suffuse, Cover, Match, and Swallow[7,8]

Wŭ, Yu-Xiang

Suffuse: Suffuse is to transport the Qi from my body to the opponent's Jin, so (he is) unable to move.

敷： 敷者，運氣于己身，敷布彼勁之上，使不得
動也。

When you learn Taijiquan, not only are you learning the forms, but you are also learning to store the Qi to an abundant level. When this Qi is transported into your body and manifested physically, the Jin can be so strong that your opponent cannot defeat you easily. When you are in a situation, if you can suffuse the Qi from your body to your opponent's body, you will be able to feel (listen) the opponent's intention. That means your Qi covers you and your opponent's body but is controlled by only you. Once you have reached this level, you will easily sense even the slightest move from your opponent. In this case, even before he manifests his Jin to your body, you have already totally controlled him. This sentence emphasizes the importance of Guardian Qi (Wei Qi, 衛氣) which envelops your body. It is through this Qi that you can feel or sense. Wei Qi is the Qi cloud on the surface of your body for defending against negative influences. When this Qi is strong, you will not catch cold easily, and your skin sensitivity will increase.

Cover: Cover, is to use the Qi to cover of the opponent's coming place (Jin manifestation origin).

四字密訣：敷、蓋、對、吞 武禹襄

蓋： 蓋者，以氣蓋彼來處也。

Once you can spread your Qi to the opponent's body and sense his intention, use your mind to lead the Qi to the emergence point for your opponent's intended action. When you can sense this intention before it is manifested, it is called "reaching to enlightenment" in Taijiquan practice. Cover is to use the mind to lead the Qi, to the place where the action is going to be. In other words, focusing all of your attention on that place. Once your attention is there, your Qi will be led there.

Match: Match, is to use the Qi to match the opponent's coming place (Jin manifestation origin). Recognize precisely the target and then go.

對： 對者，以氣對彼來處，認定准頭而去也。

Once you can sense your opponent's intention, if your opponent's Qi is also strong to match you, then it will be hard for you to control him. In this case, you must adjust to handle the situation. You must pay attention to the opponent's attack and correspond to (i.e., match) it precisely. When you do have an opportunity, do not hesitate to attack the target immediately and accurately.

Swallow: Swallow is to use the Qi to swallow fully and lead (it) into neutralization.

吞： 吞者，以氣全吞而入于化也。

Swallow can be interpreted as "yield" in Taijiquan. That means if the coming attack is strong and fast, you should yield. When your mind is on yielding, you are defensive, and this allows your opponent's Qi and physical action to come in, but under your control (i.e., swallow). Only then are you able to lead it into neutralization. In fact, the above four words are a reiteration of the listen, follow, and adhere Jins.

Song of Pulling the Bow to Store the Jin[7]

Wŭ, Yu-Xiang

蓄勁張弓歌 武禹襄

Body is bow body and the Jin is (emitted) as an arrow, adhere and follow to lead the power in spiral (i.e., coil).

身是弓身勁似箭，粘隨引進走螺旋；

In Chinese martial arts, it is commonly recognized that there are six bows found in the human body. These bows are able to store the Jin and then manifest it. The torso is normally considered constructed from the two biggest bows; the spine and chest. These two bows have the most powerful muscles/tendons, which are able to store significant Jin. Other than these two bows, the two arms and two legs are considered to be four other bows. Often, the torso is considered to be one bow, since the spinal bow and the chest bow are frequently coordinated with each other without separation.

The torso is considered most important in order to store Jin potentiality and manifest it powerfully. Even though the power is emitted from the torso, you must still observe the important criteria of Taijiquan practice, adhere, follow, and coil to neutralize incoming power.

Kicking, striking, Na (i.e., Qin Na), and wrestling, do not struggle with Li (i.e., muscular force). When (the arrow) leaves the string, do not miss the cavity.

踢打拿跌不鬥力，離弦莫叫與穴偏。

Generally, there are four categories of fighting techniques that are required for any martial style to have an effective battle. These four categories are: kicking (Ti, 踢), hand striking (Da, 打), Qin Na (擒拿) (i.e., joint control), and wrestling (Shuai, 摔). Technically speaking, wrestling is designed for use against kicking and striking, Qin Na is trained to counter grabbing and against wrestling, and kicking and striking are able to subdue Qin Na. These four categories mutually support and conquer each other and become a perfect style.

It is the same in Taijiquan, which also requires these four categories. However, when Taijiquan applies the four categories of techniques, the way to manifest power is very different. Taijiquan is classified as a soft style, and its Jin acts like a soft whip. Therefore, muscular power or force is generally avoided. Without muscular power, you must concentrate the whip-like power to a cavity, so that it can be penetrating and shocking to the internal organs. It is said: Taijiquan power is sharp and deep. This means the power is concentrated at the cavities. Therefore, the accuracy of striking and the way of manifesting soft Jin must be correct.

Internal and external mutually coordinate (relying on) the line in the tube. Up, down, left, and right, the central Qi is the first concern.

內外相合管中線，上下左右中氣先；

Jin has been classified into internal Jin (Nei Jin, 內勁) and external Jin (Wai Jin, 外勁). Internal Jin is learning how to build up the Qi at the Lower Dan Tian to an abundant level and also how to lead the Qi, with coordination of breathing, to the desired physical zone (e.g., arms and legs) for power manifestation. External Jin is learning how to construct an effective posture to store the Jin, and also how to emit the Jin so stored. When Jin is manifested powerfully, you must have both internal Jin and external Jin, otherwise, the Jin manifested will be shallow and weak. The coordination of internal and external relies on the spine in the torso. The Qi is led along the spine upward (i.e., Governing Vessel, Du Mai, 督脈) and then spread to the arms from the upper back (Dazhui, Gv-14, 大椎). This is a martial Grand Circulation (Da Zhou Tian, 大周天), which allows you to lead the Qi from the Mingmen (Gv-4)(命門) cavity to the upper limbs, to energize the limbs to the most efficient power. In addition, the torso is the main bow that stores the Jin in posture. That is why it is said, both external and internal rely on the torso.

In order to be soft, you cannot use muscular strength. It does not matter which direction you are moving, first is your mind to lead the Qi, and the physical actions follow.

Single body with five bows are ready to emit, spread, cover, match, and swallow should be pondered and studied profoundly.

一身五弓備蓄發，敷蓋對吞仔細研。

A body has five bows (torso counts as one)(Wu Gong, 五弓), and if you are skillful in storing the Jin, they can react at any time and any place. Even if you know how to store the Jin in these five bows, you must also learn and practice the four key techniques of spread, cover, match, and swallow, which were discussed in the previous documents.

Body Maneuver[7]

Wŭ, Yu-Xiang

身法 武禹襄

> Draw in the chest, stretch the back, wrap the inner thighs, protect the hips, lift the anus, hanging the crotch, prance exchange (i.e., nimbly step and jump), dodge and battle, loosing shoulders, and sunken elbow.
>
> 涵〔含〕胸、拔背、裹襠、護臀、提頂、吊襠、騰挪、閃戰、鬆肩、沉肘。

Swallow the chest is to yield and allow the opponent's power to come in, so you can lead and further neutralize. Stretch the back is when you are yielding, you are also storing the Jin in the torso's arcing posture. In order to have a firm root, the inner thigh area (Kua, 胯 or Dang, 襠) must be loose and firm. The hip area must be protected, since if your opponent can reach your hip area with the techniques of Kao (靠)(i.e., bump), you will be uprooted and lose your balance. This will allow your opponent to have an opportunity to attack you.

When Qi is stored at the Lower Dan Tian, the Huiyin (Co-1) (會陰) cavity or the anus should be lifted gently. This will allow you to lead the Qi to the Lower Dan Tian and firm your center. Hanging the crotch means to lead the bottom of the torso downward. This will firm your root and settle your foundation. When you move around, you are agile and alive. When this happens, you can dodge the incoming attack and respond offense with an effective defense. In addition to the above keys, you must also remember to sink your elbows and drop your shoulders. When you are doing so, your arms will have a root and the correct postures of storing Jin, and will then manifest it efficiently.

Thesis of Interpreting the Origin[7]

Wŭ, Cheng-Qing

[Movements]: "When (it) moves, then (it) divides, when (it is) calm, it unites." "Dividing is the dividing of Yin and Yang, and unification is the unification of Yin and Yang. The appearance of Taijiquan is as such. Dividing and unifying are all applied to myself. "The opponent does not know me, only I know the opponent." This means the Understanding Jin. After long time of pondering then will comprehend automatically.

《動》： "動之則分，靜之則合。" 分為陰陽之分，合為陰陽之合，太極之形如此：分合皆謂己而言。 "人不知我，我獨知人" ，懂勁之謂也，揣摩日久自悉矣。

This paragraph is talking about the movements of Taijiquan. When you are calm and still, it is the state of Wuji (無極)(i.e., no extremity). Once the movement is initiated, Yin and Yang divide, and when the movement ceases, Yin and Yang are re-united into the Wuji state. The original theory and concept of Taijiquan is based on this root.

In Wang, Zong-Yue's classic, it is stated: "What is Taiji? It is generated from Wuji, and is a pivotal function of movement and stillness. It is the mother of Yin and Yang. When it moves, it divides. At rest it reunites." From this statement, we can see Taiji is not Wuji, since it originates from Wuji. Taiji is also not Yin and Yang, since it is the mother of Yin and Yang. From this, you can see Taiji is the "motive force" or "driving power" of the division and re-unification. When this concept is applied to Taijiquan (i.e., martial arts with Taiji theory), then Taiji is the "mind," "idea," or "thinking." This is simply because in Taijiquan, it is the mind which drives the division and re-unification. Therefore, this mind is called the "Dao" (道) of Taijiquan. Mind is unlimited and the "grand ultimate."

Therefore, when the division and re-unification of Yin and Yang are applied, they all apply to ourselves. Because it is our minds which play the main role in Taijiquan applications. Once you can manifest your mind into physical action through feeling (i.e., Listening Jin) proficiently, you will have reached the stage of knowing yourself and also your opponent. In this case, you have grasped the key to Understanding Jin (i.e., knowing your Jin and opponent's Jin).

———————

[Leading]: "(When) lead (the coming force) to enter the emptiness, unite and then immediately emit," "(Use) four ounces to repel one thousand pounds." Unification means repelling. If (one) can comprehend this word, (then) he is the one born to wisdom.

《引》：〝引進落空合即出〞，〝四兩撥千斤〞，
合即撥也，此字能悟，真夙慧者也。

Another key concern when practicing Taijiquan is learning how to lead the incoming force into emptiness, instead of resisting it. If you do not know how to lead, then you are using force against force. When this happens, the techniques will be clumsy and the movements will be stagnant. In order to lead, your mind must first unite with your opponent's mind. Naturally, you must first be able to understand the opponent's Jin, otherwise, you will not be able to unite with the incoming force. Therefore, these unifications of your mind and the opponent's mind, as well as your force and the opponent's force are the first step to leading and repelling. Only then are you able to use only four ounces to repel one thousand pounds. Once you have neutralized the incoming force, immediately emit your Jin without hesitation. If you can comprehend the meaning of the word unification, then you have grasped the crucial key to leading and neutralization.

———————

Those who practice Taijiquan must know Yin and Yang, be able to discriminate the insubstantial and the substantial, and know advancing and retreating. When there is an advance, there is a retreating. When there is a retreating, it is advancing. Within retreating, there is a hidden maneuver of advancing. Within this, it must have (the function) of turning and unification.

夫練太極拳者須知陰陽，辨識虛實明，然後知進退，固是進中有退，退仍是進，退中隱有進機，此中須有轉合。

In order to advance and retreat, you must first be able to discriminate the Yin and Yang during the technique exchange with your opponent. However, you should also understand that even if you are advancing, you must be ready for retreating. Conversely, when you are retreating, you are setting up a new strategy for advancing. It is just like the Taiji Yin and Yang symbol. There is some Yang within the Yin and there is some Yin within the Yang. Only then are you able to move with life. You can then change your techniques skillfully, and unite your thoughts with your opponent's.

The character of the body's (posture) must have: the insubstantial energy (i.e., Jin) leads the head up, stretching the back and draw in the chest (i.e., arc the chest), Qi is sunk to the Dan Tian, wrapping the inner thighs and protecting the hips. The Spirit of Vitality must be raised, then the entire body will be able to turn as you wish, two hands are able to support the eight directions, and (techniques are) alive as cart wheels. When encountering (the opponent), there is no enemy (can match you).

身法要有虛領頂勁，拔背含胸，氣沉丹田，裏襠護
臀。精神總要提起，則周身旋轉自如，兩手支撐八
面，活似車輪，所向無敵。

This paragraph is talking about the body's posture. The first and the most important requirement in Taijiquan practice is to keep the body upright, relaxed, loose, and the head as though it were suspended from the top. This will provide you with balance, comfort, and a natural feeling of being centered. Without this feeling, you will not establish a firm root. Next, in order to store the Jin in the body, you must know how to draw in your chest and arc your back. Your torso is constructed with two bows—the chest and the spine. From these two bows the Peng Jin (掤勁)(i.e., Wardoff Jin) is commonly manifested. From Peng Jin, you can yield and store the Jin for further actions. However, you must also be concerned with another important factor. The internal side (i.e., the Yin side) of Taijiquan training, which supports external physical strength, is the Qi. Qi should be sunken and built up abundantly in the Lower Dan Tian. This will provide you with the energy required for the physical action. The physical body is like a car while the Qi is like the energy generated from fuel. If you wish your car to have a powerful potential performance, you must first use a good fuel, which can provide you with abundant, clean energy.

In order to have a firm root, the inner thighs should be firmed (i.e., wrapped) and the hips should be tucked in (i.e., protected). When these areas are firmed and steady, you will have built up a solid foundation for the root, to support the upper body's action. However, the most important factor that affects the efficiency and effectiveness of all Taijiquan activities is your Spirit. When your Spirit is high and alert, you will be in a higher mental state, which could provide you with a natural and controllable situation. The body will be alive and agile. When this happens, your two hands are so skillful, and able to handle any situation from any direction. Once you have fulfilled all of the above requirements, you will find no enemy who can match you.

When the opponent's Jin is just coming and not yet emitted, I immediately strike. This is called "strike the oppressive Jin"; when the opponent's Jin has already come, and I have already been waiting, once (the opponent's Jin has) reached my body, I strike immediately. When the opponent's power has entered the emptiness and is going to change (his) Jin, I follow (his retreating) and strike, this is called "strike the returning Jin." Experience the above (key words) and ponder carefully, (soon it will) follow (your) wish and reach the enlightenment naturally.

人勁方來，未能發出，我即打去，此謂〝打悶勁〞；人勁已來，我早靜待，著身即便打去，人已落空，欲將換勁，我隨之打去，此謂〝打回勁〞。由此體驗，留心揣摩，自然從心所欲階及神明矣。

During combat situations, the best timing for attack is when your opponent is just initiating an attack. It is said: "the opponent does not move, I do not move; the opponent moves slightly, I move first." When this happens, your opponent's Yi (i.e., mind) has already formed and the action has just began. If you suddenly attack at this time, you will have a great chance of success. If you strike with this timing, it is called "to strike the oppressive Jin."

However, what if your reaction is too slow to catch the above timing, and your opponent has already emitted his Jin toward you? In this case, if you were waiting for this attack, you have prepared for it. You can then neutralize the incoming force when first touched, and immediately attack him. However, if at this time your opponent realizes his Jin has been neutralized, he will start to pull back his attack. You should take this opportunity to follow his retreating and attack. This is called "strike the returning Jin."

In combat, the timing of interception and counter-attack is a crucial key to effectiveness for the techniques. However, you must spend a long time training and pondering. Once you have gained a lot of combat experience, you will be able to catch the correct timing and react naturally.

"Left heaviness," "right heaviness," "upward," "downward," "advancing," "retreating," are talking about the opponent. "Left insubstantial," "right disappearance," "higher," "deeper," "longer," "more urgent," are talking about yourself and also talking about the opponent. Insubstantial, disappearing, higher, deeper, are felt by the opponent (and are caused) from my leading (the coming Jin) into emptiness. "When retreating, then it is more urgent," is to force (the opponent) into a situation of no position for retreating, is (as urgent as) reining the horse near the edge of the cliff. If (the opponent) does not have Understanding Jin, (he) is unable to get away. This is what is said about upward, downward, left, right, advance, and retreat.

"左重"、"右重"、"仰之"、"俯之"、"進之"、"退之",是謂人也。"左虛"、"右杳"、"彌高"、"彌深"、"愈長"、"愈促",是謂己亦謂人也。虛、杳、高、深是人覺如此,我引彼落空也。"退之則愈促",迫無容身之地,如懸崖勒馬,非懂勁不能走也。此六句上、下、左、右、前、後之謂是矣。

When my opponent generates heaviness (i.e., pressure) on my left or right hand side, my left or right become insubstantial and lead the coming force into emptiness. When the opponent moves my force upward or downward, I initiate my Growing Jin (Zhang Jin, 長勁) and make him feel my force is higher and deeper. When the opponent advances or retreats, I continue to lead his advancing toward me while I am retreating. This will make him feel longer and beyond his reach. However, when he retreats, I advance aggressively and make him feel urgent. It is just like he is riding a horse near the edge of a cliff. If he is not knowledgeable and skillful in Understanding Jin, he will not be able to handle the situation.

"(When) sunken to the side, then follow. (When) double weighting, then stagnant." This is to compare with (the saying) "alive as the cart wheel." It is talking about myself. (When) this is sunken in one side, then turn. (If) both sides are weighted, then stagnant. If not allowing the double weighting, then will not be controlled. This is talking about the sickness (i.e., mistakes) of myself. When it is stiff, then it will become as such (i.e., double weighting). When it is soft, then follow. Follow then give up myself and follow the opponent. (In this case, it) will not be glued on the post (i.e., stiff) and stagnant.

〝偏沉則隨，雙重則滯〞，是比〝活似車輪〞而言，乃己之謂。一邊沉則轉，兩邊重則滯，不使雙重，即不為制矣！是言己之病也。硬則如此，軟則隨，隨則舍己從人，不為膠柱鼓瑟矣！

When the opponent puts pressure on either side of my body, I can simply turn and neutralize the incoming force easily. However, if the opponent applies pressure on both sides of my body, and if I resist in both sides, it is called "double-weighting" and means to put weight on the weight. In this case, simply sink one side and then turn the body to neutralize the pressure. The technique must be applied skillfully and in an alive manner, like the rotation of a cartwheel. If you do not know the trick to the neutralization, you will be double-weighted and controlled by your opponent. Once you are double-weighting, you will be stiff and your skill will be stagnant.

Thesis of the Fist[7]

Wǔ, Cheng-Qing

When learn the striking hands (i.e., sparring) at the beginning, first learn Rollback (Lu), Push (An), and Elbow (Zhou). This is when (I) use rollback, the opponent uses the elbow, when (I) use push, the opponent uses rollback, two persons are the same, repeat with cycle, and is called "old three matching." After this, high posture and low posture, gradually increase the number, where the top or the bottom of the entire body is attacked, where (I) intercept (the coming attacks). The body turns following the Jin (my Jin). Talk about the internal Gong instead of the external appearance.

初學打手，先學攦、按、肘。此用攦彼用肘，此用
按彼用攦，二人一樣，循環往復，周而復始，謂之
〝老三著〞。以後高勢低勢漸漸加多，周身上下打
著何處，何處接應，身隨勁〔己之勁〕轉，論內功
不論外形。

To learn Taiji sparring, you should first learn three basic Taiji moving patterns: Rollback (Lu, 攦), Push (An, 按), and Elbow (Zhou, 肘). From these basic patterns, you can grasp the basic keys of listening, following, sticking, and adhering. In this practice, the Elbow is used against rollback and rollback is used against push. It is called "old three matching." You should practice both high and low postures and gradually increase the number of repetitions. When you practice, at the beginning, pay attention to the correct postures. Next, learn to generate the Jin from the legs, directed by the waist, and then manifested in the hands. Once you have the mind of manifesting the Jin, the way you use the waist to direct the Jin is crucial. Once the mind is generated, the Qi is led. Without external coordination, the Jin cannot be manifested efficiently.

This is the way to train striking hands (i.e., sparring). When train until (the stage of) purely skillful, (you are) able to lead the (opponent's) Jin into emptiness, unify (your Jin) and emit, then the art is accomplished. However, if not knowing Understanding Jin (i.e., your Jin and the opponent's Jin), (you will) not be able to know how the opponent's Jin is coming and how to use your Jin to lead.

此打手磨練之法，練到純熟時，能引勁〔人之勁〕
落空合即出，則藝業成矣。然非懂勁〔此勁字兼言
人、己之勁〕不能知人勁怎樣來，己之勁當怎樣引
進。

The way of reaching high levels of skill is through constant practice. The more you practice, the better you will be and naturally, the more skillfully and efficiently the techniques can be executed. The goal of this practice is to gain the skills of Listening Jin and Understanding Jin. From these two Jins, you will be able to use four ounces to neutralize one thousand pounds. That means to lead the opponent's Jin into emptiness. Once you have neutralized the incoming Jin, you can emit your Jin. In order to achieve this skill, you must know how to stick and adhere to the incoming Jin, unify with it and then lead it away.

The marvelous trick within must be comprehended from the (deep) heart. (This) cannot (only) be passed down orally. (When) the heart knows, then the body will know. (When) the body knows, it is better than (only) the heart knows. (Once you) can comprehend from the heart and from the body (i.e., apply to the body), the Jin can be agile in movement. (If one) only knows in the heart, still (he) cannot apply it (in the body). Only when known by the body (i.e., applied), then is Understanding Jin. Understanding Jin is really not easy.

此中巧妙必須心悟，不能口授。心知方能身知，身
知勝于心知：悟于心知身知，勁乃靈動，徒心知尚
不應用，到得身知方為懂勁。懂勁詢不易也。

Although the theory is simple and the principles of practice are straightforward, there are still not too many people who are able to apply these skills in sparring. The reason for this is simply that comprehension is not deep and profound. Just knowing the theory and principles but being unable to apply them into action is not really understanding. Those who really comprehend Understanding Jin should be able to apply the theory and principles into action skillfully and efficiently.

Song of Striking Hands[7]

Wǔ, Cheng-Qing

打手歌 武澄清

Be serious in Wardoff (Peng), Rollback (Lu), Press (Ji),
and Push (An), Pluck (Cai), Split (Lie), Elbow (Zhou),
and Bump (Kao), follow the bending and extending.

掤攦擠按須認真，採挒肘靠就曲伸。

Among the thirteen postures of Taijiquan, the first four: Wardoff,
Rollback, Press, and Push, must be studied and practiced seriously. If
you can comprehend these four major training areas, you will have
grasped the basic essence of Taijiquan practice. In addition to these
four, Pluck, Split, Elbow, and Bump are four assisting techniques. In
order to store and emit Jin in these techniques, you should always
remember the key to bending (storing) and emitting (extending).

Advance (Jin), Retreat (Tui), Beware of the Left (Gu),
Look to the Right (Pan), and also Central Equilibrium
(Zhong Ding), adhere to connect and follow, the
insubstantial and substantial are discriminated.

進退顧盼與中定，粘連依隨虛實分；

Other than the above eight basic Jin patterns, Taijiquan also
includes five strategic movements: Advance (Jin, 進), Retreat (Tui, 退),
Beware of the Left (Gu, 顧), Look to the Right (Pan, 盼), and also
Central Equilibrium (Zhong Ding, 中定). In total there are thirteen
postures or basic patterns. In order to perform all of these patterns
effectively, you must learn how to listen (i.e., skin feeling), adhere to
connect, and also how to follow the opponent's force. In addition,

you must be able to distinguish the Yin and Yang aspects of Taijiquan applications. Only then can you understand the strategy of insubstantial and substantial.

Hands and feet mutually follow each other and integrate with the waist and the legs. Lead (the coming force) into the emptiness, (its applications) is marvelous and splendid.

手足相隨腰腿整，引進落空妙如神，

In Taijiquan practice, the top should be coordinated with the bottom. That means the arms are coordinating with the legs, the wrists are coordinating with the ankles, the elbows are coordinating with the knees, and the shoulders are coordinating with the hips. Moreover, the internal (i.e., mind, Qi, and breathing) must coordinate with the external physical movements. The legs are Yin and the power's manifestation at the arms is Yang. The internal aspect of Qi storage and circulation is Yin while the external aspect of power manifestation is Yang. Once you can comprehend and discriminate such Yin and Yang clearly, and will also know how to use the waist to control and direct the movement (i.e., central equilibrium), then you have grasped the essential key to neutralization and can lead the incoming force into emptiness. Taijiquan can be so marvelous and splendid simply because it does not use force against force.

It does not matter if the opponent uses giant power to strike forward, (simply) use the four ounces to lead the movement and repel the thousand pounds.

任他巨力向前打，牽動四兩撥千斤。

Once you can lead the incoming force into the emptiness, then you can use only four ounces to neutralize one thousand pounds.

This song talks about the foundation of Taijiquan in thirteen postures (or moving patterns). Next, it emphasizes the importance of the upper body and lower body's coordination, and the entire body acting as one single unit. All of the coordination and connection in the upper and lower body relies on how well you can use the waist to harmoniously control the movements. Once you can do so, you will have learned the most crucial key to Taijiquan practice, neutralizing the incoming force using only slight power.

A Postscript[7]

Wǔ, Cheng-Qing

跋

武澄清

(For) the scholarship of Taijiquan, the thesis written by Wang, Zong-Yue is the real essence. Its techniques use the softness and bend as the body (i.e., main techniques) and use the hardness and straight as the applications. It is because when the giant force arrives, without softness and bend cannot neutralize (the force) skillfully. Once the (coming) is neutralized, without hardness and straight, (the Jin) cannot be manifested to far (distance). Therefore, it is said: "Search for the straight within the bend, store and then emit."

太極拳學，王宗岳論之精矣！其術以柔曲為體，以剛直為用。蓋巨力之至，非柔曲不能化之靈，彼力既化，非剛直不能放之遠，故曰：「曲中求直，蓄而後發。」

According to the author, Master Wang, Zong-Yue's Taijiquan thesis can be the representative essence and root of Taijiquan. What this thesis has discussed is how to use the softness and "bend" (i.e., round) against strong incoming force. Once the incoming force has been neutralized, in order to reach far and manifest the Jin effectively, the emitting Jin must be strong and straight forward. That means, within the softness, there is a hardness, and within the hardness, there is a softness. Within the bending, there is a straightness, and within the straight, there is a bending.

When practicing these techniques, (the key) is that the Qi is sunk at the Dan Tian. It is purely executed with the Spirit, and does not depend on the clumsy post-heaven force. When defending against the enemy to win (the battle), it is as doing nothing (i.e., be natural). Though (the techniques are) skillful, the ultimate Dao (i.e., theory and principle) is existing. Lao Zi said: "If wish to take, must give (first)." The original classic said: "(When) the left is heavy then the left (becomes) insubstantial, (when) the right is heavy, then the right disappears," that means the opponent takes and I give. Juang Zi said: "(If one is) able to keep in the ring (i.e., grasp the keys), (one) can respond (the situations) without limitation." It is also said "the Qi is like a cart wheel, transport the Qi as in a nine curved pearl." That means (you have) kept in the ring. Therefore, the technique of "specialize the Qi in the softness" is consistent with Dao family. Without few ten years of pure Gong, (one will) not be able to use it skillfully.

練習此術，在氣沉丹田，純以神行，不尚後天之拙
力；而御敵制勝，如行所無事，雖甚巧而有至道存
焉。老子曰：〝若欲取之，必固與之。〞原譜所謂
〝左重則左虛，右重則右杳〞，即人取我與之意。
莊子曰：〝得其環中，以應無窮〞。所謂氣如車輪
，行氣如九曲珠，即得其環中之意也。故其術〝專
氣致柔〞，蓋合于道家，非數十年純功，不能用之
精巧。

All of the techniques are manifested through Jin. Jin is the martial power which originates from the Yi (i.e., mind). From this mind, the Qi is led to the places of the body and the Jin is manifested. The strength of the Qi depends on how abundantly the Qi has been stored in the Lower Dan Tian. When the Qi is full in the Lower Dan Tian, and if you know how to use reverse abdominal breathing to sink the Qi there (to balance the upward Qi), and you can manifest it to the hands, the power can be so strong. While you are doing this, you should also raise up the Spirit of Vitality. When the Spirit is high, the power and techniques can be executed efficiently. Therefore, Taijiquan's power is not the same as many external martial styles which pay more attention to external muscular power.

At the beginning of executing your techniques, you must first use your mind to regulate the body, the breathing, the mind, the Qi, and the Spirit. However, after you have practiced for a long period of time, all of the required factors of manifesting the Jin in the techniques have become so natural that you will be in the stage of "the fight of no fight." This means your reaction is so natural that your mind does not have to react. When this happens, you have reached the "Dao" of fighting.

The crucial key to Taijiquan is to give first so you can take. This means you first must follow the opponent's desire by listening (i.e., skin feeling) and following. Only then can you lead his incoming force into emptiness. Once his force has been neutralized, then you can attack. Therefore, when the opponent puts pressure or force onto either side of my body, I simply make the attacked area insubstantial until it disappears. Once I am able to catch this trick, then I can stay soft and transport my Qi freely and smoothly.

This fist (i.e., style) pays attention in the emptiness and insubstantial, and avoids the double weighting. Isn't this what Lao Zi said?: "Insubstantial but not giving up, (when) moving, the more (action) is manifested." The Jin of Taiji can be broken, (but) the Yi (i.e., wisdom mind) is not broken. Isn't this what Lao Zi said?: "Soft and slender as existing." Taiji follows to bend and then to extend, the Yi (wisdom mind) is ahead the opponent's. Isn't this what Lao Zi said?: "(When) receiving without seeing its head and (when) following without seeing its tail." Therefore, I say if (one) wishes to see these tricks, it is in Taiji's thirteen postures.

此拳貴空虛忌雙重，非老子之〝虛而不屈，動而愈出〞者乎！太極之勁斷意不斷，非老子之〝綿綿若存〞者乎！太極之隨曲就伸，意在人先，非老子之〝迎而不見其首，隨之不見其後〞者乎！故吾謂有欲以觀其竅者，即太極之十三勢也。

Taijiquan emphasizes the skills of leading the opponent's force into emptiness and avoiding mutual resistance. Double weighting means that when the opponent places some weight (i.e., force) on me, I respond with weight (i.e., force). Even if you are leading the opponent's force into emptiness and you are in the insubstantial condition, you are not giving up or giving in. Your listening and following is only a neutralization strategy, and is a setup for future attack. To make this strategy effective, the mind is always there, ahead of the Jin's manifestation. In this case, you are soft yet your mind is controlling the entire situation. Once you have grasped this trick, then your opponent will not be able to figure out from where and how your power is coming, and where and how it goes. Your opponent does not know you and you know your opponent. Application of these principles will allow you to control the entire confrontation.

Thesis of Taijiquan[13]

Wŭ, Ru-Qing

太極拳論 武汝清

The fist (i.e., style) named as Taijiquan, (is rooted with) Yin-Yang and insubstantial-substantial. (If) Yin and Yang is clear (i.e., understood), then (can) know advance and retreating. Even advance is for advance, there is retreating within advancing. (When) stepping backward, it is still advance, because within the retreating, there is an intention of advance hidden. Among all of these variations, the keys are: (using the) insubstantial Jin (energy) to lead the head upward and stretching the back and containing the chest, then the Spirit of Vitality can raise up. Qi is sunk at the Dan Tian and wrapping the inner thighs and also protecting the hips, then (it is) easy to handle (the situations). Elbow should bend properly. (When) bent and able to extend, then there is an advantage in supporting (the Jin's manifestation) and gaining advantageous position. The knees should store (the Jin). (When) store and can emit, then there is power in emitting the Jin. When exchanging hands with opponent (i.e., sparring), the hands must first feel the force. Only listen the opponent's Jin, be sure (to) follow the opponent and do not follow yourself. Also (you) must be sure that (you) know the opponent and do not let the opponent know you.

夫拳名太極者，陰陽虛實也。陰陽明然後知進退，
進故是進，進中有退，步退仍是進，退中隱有進機
。此中轉關，在於虛領頂勁，而拔背含胸，則精神
提得起；氣沉丹田而裹襠護臀，則周旋便捷。肘宜
曲，曲而能伸，則支撐得勢。膝宜蓄，蓄而能發，
則發勁有力。至與人交手，手先著力，只聽人勁，
務要由人，不要由己；務要知人，不要使人知己。

Taijiquan was created based on the theory of Taiji (i.e., Grand Ultimate). Taiji theory was first discovered in the book Yi Jing (Book of Changes, 易經, 1122 B.C.). From this Taiji theory, the Yin and Yang concepts are derived. When Yin and Yang concepts are applied to Taijiquan martial arts, it means insubstantial and substantial. Taiji and Yin-Yang theory have therefore become the root of Taijiquan development.

When you practice Taijiquan, you should always keep Yin and Yang concepts in your mind and apply them into your thinking and action. Only then can you understand the skills of advancing and retreating. When there is an advance, you should always be conservative and leave some space for retreating. Naturally, when you are retreating, you are in fact setting up an opportunity for advancing.

To make all of this theory work, the head must be upright and the Spirit of Vitality must be raised. In order to manifest Peng Jin (i.e., the first Taijiquan posture) effectively, the back should be arced and the chest should be contained. The Qi is abundant and sunk to the Lower Dan Tian. In order to keep the posture firm and rooted, the inner thighs should be turned inward (i.e., wrapped) and the hips should be locked in (i.e., protected). Once you have a firm root, you can use your waist to direct the power easily and skillfully. Elbows should be bent (i.e., sink the elbow), then the arms are connected (i.e., rooted) to the body. When this happens, the Jin manifested will be powerful and have a firm foundation. Since the power is generated from the legs, whenever it is possible, keep your legs bent so that the power can be emitted anytime.

Once you are attacked, remember listening and following first. Only then can you lead the incoming force into emptiness. If you resist, your opponent will know your intention immediately. In this case, you are in a double-weighting situation. However, if you are soft and follow the opponent's force, you will be able to neutralize the incoming power. When this happens, you will know your opponent but your opponent will not know you.

If (you) know the opponent, then up and down, advance and retreat, and left and right, (you) naturally will be able to lead the (incoming force) into the emptiness. The key trick in this is on the shoulders' relaxation, controlled by the waist, rooted on the feet, but listening the order in the heart (i.e., respond with natural feeling). Once move, there is no place does not move, when calm, there is no place does not calm. The top and the bottom (are unified) with one Qi. It is what is said, standing as the scale (i.e., balanced) and alive like a cart wheel. Support the eight directions and there is no match when encountering (the opponent).

知人則上下前後左右自能引進落空，則人背我順。
此中轉關在乎鬆肩，主宰于腰，立根在腳，但聽命
于心。一動無有不動，一靜無有不靜。上下一氣，
即所謂立如秤準，活似車輪，支撐八面，所向無敵
。

If you can feel and sense the opponent's intention and his incoming force, you can lead them into emptiness. However, to make this neutralization work, you must sink the shoulders and keep them soft. Any slight movement is directed by the waist, and the legs must be firmly rooted, reacting to the situation naturally. Only then will your entire body act as one unit. When it moves, the entire body moves, and when it is calm, the entire body is calm. When you are in this state, you can respond both mentally and physically.

(When) the opponent's Jin is forming and not yet able to be emitted, I immediately strike to attack, it is called "striking the nascent Jin." (When) the opponent's Jin has already come and I am waiting calmly, once reaching (my) body, immediately I strike and attack, it is called "striking the coming Jin." (When) the opponent's Jin has already been led and entered the emptiness, and (he) is going to change the Jin, I follow (his retreating) and strike, it is called "striking the returning Jin." From this to experience and ponder cautiously, (you will) be able to fulfill (your) wish and reach enlightenment gradually.

人勁將來，未能發出，我即打去，謂之〝打悶勁〞。人勁已來，我早靜待，著身即便打去，所謂〝打來勁〞。人勁已落空，將欲換勁，我隨打去，此謂〝打回勁〞。由此體驗，留心揣摩，自能從心所欲，階及神明矣。

There are three attacking timings in a fight. The first is when the opponent's Yi (i.e., intention) has already revealed itself, but before the Jin has been emitted. At this time, if you attack suddenly, you can suppress his intention and successfully execute your attack. This is because at this time, your opponent's mind is on attacking rather than defense. Therefore, it is said: "When the opponent slightly moves, I move first."

The second timing is when the opponent's Jin is being emitted, but you are prepared for it and are expecting it. As his Jin reaches your body, lead it to emptiness and immediately attack. To make this timing effective, you must know how to neutralize the incoming power skillfully.

The third timing is when the opponent's Jin has already been emitted, but has lost its purpose due to your dodging or neutralization, and he is pulling back to change to a new strategy, by emitting another Jin based technique. If you attack while he is withdrawing, often you can reach him as well.

Among the three timings, the first is the most difficult simply because you must be able to perceive the opponent's intention even before he manifests it. When you reach this stage, you have touched enlightenment in fighting. The second timing is the second most difficult. You must be skillful in listening, following, sticking, and adhering so you can neutralize the incoming Jin, but also follow with your own attack. This is the most commonly used of the timings. The last timing, though also commonly used, can often be dissolved easily by the opponent. This is because when the opponent is withdrawing, he is already mentally prepared for your attack.

The Secret of Withdraw and Release[1,6-8]

Li, Yi-Yu

撤放密訣

李亦畬

First Saying: Deflect and open opponent's body and borrow opponent's Li (strength). Within there is the word of agility.

一曰擎，擎開彼身借彼力，中有靈字。

Do not meet the opponent's attack head on, or try to block it with force. Let your arm touch the opponent's arm, match his speed and direction, and deflect his attack from its original direction. If the opponent throws a right punch and you deflect it to your right, his right side will be exposed. When the opponent uses strength, he will tend to be stiff. If you deflect him properly, his strength and momentum will cause him to lose balance. In this sense you are "borrowing" his strength to defeat him.

In order to make this deflection effective and skillful, you must train to be agile, as well as strong, fast and soft. Without dexterity, your deflection (i.e., neutralization) will not be effective. The way of achieving a high level of dexterity is to train listening, understanding, adhering, and following Jins.

Second Saying: Lead (opponent's power) near (my) body, Jin thereby stored. Within there is the word of condensing.

二曰引，引到身前勁始蓄，中有斂字。

When you neutralize an opponent's attack, draw him into you somewhat, and accumulate energy in your posture and Qi in your Lower Dan Tian and spine. This is just like a bow accumulating energy when it is drawn, or a spring when it is compressed. You should also inhale in order to coordinate the motion with your Qi.

The key image for leading the Qi to the Lower Dan Tian is condensing the Qi around you to the center of your body. This means to condense the Qi to the Lower Dan Tian and also to the bone marrow.

Third Saying: Relax and expand my Jin, without bends.
Within there is the word of calmness.

三曰鬆，鬆開我勁勿使屈，中有靜字。

The major difference between the Jin used in Taijiquan and the Jin of other styles is that Taiji emphasizes soft Jin, and requires significant Qi support. This makes it possible to develop the Jin to a higher level. The first step in this development is relaxation. You must relax all of your muscles so that the Qi can flow wherever you want it to go, without any hindrance. The Qi will then suffuse the muscles so that they function at peak efficiency.

When you counterattack, you relax and emit Jin the way a bow relaxes from a state of tension as it shoots an arrow. Your posture should not have any kinks or awkward bends. Thus it is said: "Relax and expand my Jin, without bends."

When you apply force with your hand, there should be a counter-force into your rear foot to balance it. The line from the hand to the rear foot should be direct, without any "bends" (awkwardness in the posture, or inward collapse) to disperse the energy. Thus it is said in Taijiquan: "Jin is straight and not curved."

In order to be relaxed, first you must be calm. Without calmness, your mind will be scattered and confused. When this happens, your body will be tight, and you will not be relaxed. Confucius said: "First, you must calm, then your mind will be steady. When your mind is steady, you will be peaceful." Once you have reached a peaceful state both mentally and physically, you can relax. Therefore, the crucial key word for relaxation is calmness.

Fourth Saying: When (I) release, the waist and the feet must be timed carefully and accurately. Within there is the word of wholeness.

四曰放，放時腰腳認端的，中有整字。

In order for the released Jin to reach its maximum level, your feet must be firmly rooted in the ground, the Jin must be generated from the legs, and the waist must control and direct it. Timing is critical in order to release your Jin effectively and efficiently. If you do not grasp the right moment to accurately express your Jin in attack or defense, it will be clumsy and inefficient, and you will miss the opportunity and lose the advantage. It is just like shooting at a moving target with a bow and arrow. The timing of the arrow's release and the accuracy of the aim are the keys to hitting the target.

When you emit your Jin, your entire body must act as one unit. From the bottom of your feet to the fingers is threaded together and acts as a soft whip. The targeting of the cavity must be accurate, and the power must be penetrating. Only then can the corresponding internal organ be shocked and the opponent defeated.

Five Key Words[1,6-8]

Li, Yi-Yu

五字訣 李亦畬

First Saying: The Xin (heart, mind) is quiet (calm). When the heart (mind) is not quiet (calm), then (I am) not concentrated on one (thing). When I lift hands, forward and backward, left and right, (I am) totally without direction (purpose). In the beginning the movements do not follow the mind. Put the heart on recognizing and experiencing. Follow the opponent's movements, follow the curve, then expand. Don't lose (him), don't resist, don't extend or withdraw by yourself. (If the) opponent has Li (power), I also have Li, but my Li is first. (If the) opponent is without power, I also am without power, however my Yi (mind) is still first. One must be careful every movement. Wherever I am in contact, there the heart (mind) must be. One must seek information from not losing and not resisting; if I do that from now on, in one year or in half a year I will then be able to apply this with my body. All of this is using Yi (the mind), not using Jin. If I practice longer and longer, then the opponent is controlled by me, and I am not controlled by the opponent.

一曰心靜。心不靜則不專一。一舉手，前後左右，全無定向，故要心靜。起初舉動，未能由己，要悉心體認，隨人所動，隨屈就伸，不丟不頂，勿自伸縮。彼有力，我亦有力，我力在先。彼無力，我亦無力，我意仍在先。要刻刻留心，挨何處，心要用在何處。須向不丟不頂中討消息；從此做去，一年半載，便能施於身，此全是用意，不是用勁，久之則人為我制，我不為人制矣。

In Taijiquan, the mind is most important and controls movement. You cannot achieve this control by asserting your will. You must "give up yourself and follow the other." Don't resist, don't lose contact. Your power and mind are first in that you lead the opponent's attack away, rather than push it away. If you always remain lightly attached to the opponent you will gradually learn to sense his intentions. When you can follow automatically, your mind will be quiet and able to control your body and the opponent.

Second Saying: The body is agile. If the body is stagnant, then (moving) forward and backward can't be at will. Therefore the body must be agile. When you lift your hands you must not have a clumsy appearance. When the opponent's power just touches my skin, my Yi (mind) is already deep into his bones. Two hands support, one Qi threading all through. (If) the left is heavy (attacked), then the left becomes insubstantial, (and) the right is gone (attacks). (If) the right is heavy, then the right becomes insubstantial and the left is gone. Qi is just like a cartwheel. Each part of the body must be mutually coordinated. If there is a place not mutually coordinated, then the body is dispersed and disordered, then you cannot gain power. (If you have) this fault, you must look to the waist and legs. First use your heart (mind) to master your body, following the opponent, not following your own will. Then the body can follow the heart. Now, you can follow your own will or follow the opponent. If you follow your own will, then stagnation. If you follow the opponent, then you are alive. If able to follow the opponent, then the top of your hand has centimeters and inches. Weigh the opponent's Jin, big or small, then you have centimeters and millimeters with no mistakes. Measure the opponent's movement, long or short, then (you will make) no errors, even by a hairsbreadth. Forward and backward, everywhere just matches (the opponent). The longer you study, then the finer your technique.

二曰身靈。身滯則進退不能自如，故要身靈。舉手
不可有呆像，彼之力方挨我皮毛，我之意已入彼骨
裡。兩手支撐，一氣貫串，左重則左虛，而右已去
，右重則右虛，而左已去。氣如車輪，週身俱要相
隨，有不相隨處，身便散亂，便不得力，其病於腰
腿求之。先以心使身，從人不從己，後身能從心，
由己仍是從人。由己則滯，從人則活。能從人，手
上便有分寸。秤彼勁之大小，分厘不錯。權來意之
長短，毫髮無差。前進後退，處處恰合，工彌久而
技彌精。

When you are light and agile and practice following for a long time, you can interpret the opponent's intentions at his lightest touch. Your two hands work together as a unit. When the opponent puts pressure on (attacks) your right side, that side becomes insubstantial (yields) and your left side has already attacked. When you can follow the opponent, then you can judge and interpret his actions and respond appropriately. The more you practice, the finer your sensitivity and control will be. It is as if your hand had a ruler or micrometer on it to measure the opponent's actions.

Third Saying: Qi condenses. When the Qi is dispersed and diffused, then it is not conserved, and the body can easily be scattered and disordered. In order to make Qi condense into the bones your exhalation and inhalation must flow agilely (smoothly). The entire body is without gap. Inhalation is storage, and exhalation is emitting. That is because inhalation lifts up naturally (the Spirit of Vitality). It can also lift (control) the opponent. (When you) exhale, then (your Qi) can sink naturally. (You) also can release (Jin) out to the opponent. That means use Yi (your mind) to move your Qi, don't use Li (strength).

TAI CHI QI AND JIN: A STRING OF PEARLS

若氣勢散漫，便無含蓄，身易散亂，務使
氣斂入脊骨，呼吸通靈。週身無間，吸為合為蓄，
呼為開為發。蓋吸則自然提得起，亦拏得人起。呼
則自然沉得下，亦放人得出，此是以意運氣，非以
力使氣也。

When your Qi is scattered about your body in an undisciplined fashion, your body will be disorganized. You must calm the mind. When you inhale, let the Qi accumulate in the Dan Tian and spine, and raise the Spirit of Vitality. When you exhale, move the Qi from the spine, to the shoulders, and out to the hands. When you exhale, the Qi is also fully sunk to the tailbone. Breathing must be unhindered and must comfortably match your actions.

Fourth Saying: Jin is integrated. The entire body's Jin, (when) trained, becomes one family (one unit). Distinguish clearly insubstantial and substantial. Emitting Jin must have root and origin. Jin begins at the foot's root, is controlled by the waist, expressed by the fingers, emitted by the spine and back. (You) must also lift the entire Spirit of Vitality. When the opponent's Jin is just about to be emitted, but is not yet emitted, my Jin already accepts it in (senses it). Just right, not late, not early. (It is) just like the skin (senses) fire. Like a spring bubbling up from the ground. Forward, backward, not the slightest scattering or confusion. Look for the straight in the curved. Store and then emit. (If you do this) then you will be able to follow the (opponent's) hands and act effectively. This is borrowing (the opponent's) Li to strike the opponent, and (using) four ounces to repel a thousand pounds.

四曰勁整。一身之勁，練成一家，分清虛實，發勁
要有根源，勁起於腳根，主宰於腰，發於脊背，形
於手指，又要提起全副精神，於彼勁將出未發之際
，我勁已接入彼勁。恰好不後不先，如皮燃火，如
泉湧出，前進後退，無絲毫散亂，曲中求直，蓄而
後發，方能隨手奏效，此借力打人，四兩撥千斤也
。

You must learn how all parts of the body contribute to the technique, what parts are heavy or active, and what parts are light or insubstantial. Jin is rooted in the feet, it originates in (is generated by) the legs, is controlled by the waist, emitted by the spine, and expressed by the hands. Raising the Spirit of Vitality allows you to have a strong root and a clear mind. Timing is crucial for effective technique. You must develop the lightness and sensitivity to respond to the opponent's attack as quickly and unconsciously as the skin responds to fire. At the first touch, or even before the touch, you know his intention and are already neutralizing him. Your movement and response must be continuous and flowing like a spring bubbling up out of the ground. You are continuously moving in curves and circles. This allows you to bend like a bow or coil like a spring and accumulate energy in your posture. You also accumulate Qi in your spine and Dan Tian. When you neutralize you curve or bend, and then you attack in a straight line. If you learn these skills you will be able to defeat your opponent easily and automatically.

Fifth Saying: Spirit condenses. All in all, (if) the above four items (are) totally acquired, it comes down to condensing Shen (Spirit). When Shen condenses, then one Qi (can be) formed, like a drum. Training Qi belongs to Shen. Qi appears agitated (i.e., abundant) and smooth. The Spirit of Vitality is threaded and concentrated. Opening and closing have numbers (degrees of fineness). Insubstantial and substantial are clearly distinguished: if the left is insubstantial, then the right is substantial; if the right is insubstantial, then the left is substantial. Insubstantial doesn't mean absolutely no Li. The appearance of Qi must have agitation and smoothness; in actuality it does not happen instantly by magic. The Spirit of Vitality should be emphasized, it must be threaded and concentrated. Li is borrowed from the opponent. Qi is emitted from the spine. How can Qi come from the spine? (When) Qi sinks downward from the two shoulders, condenses into the bones of the spine, concentrates at the waist (Dan Tian), this Qi from the top to the bottom is called closing. From the waist, appearing in the bones of the spine, then spreading to the shoulders, appearing in the fingers, this Qi from the bottom to the top is called opening. Closing means to draw in, opening means to release. If able to understand opening and closing, then (you) know Yin and Yang. When you understand these steps, then (if you) practice one day, your technique is refined one day. (Then you) gradually approach (the point) where you can not but achieve what you want.

五曰神聚。上四者俱備，總歸神聚，神聚則一氣鼓鑄，練氣歸神，氣勢騰挪，精神貫注，開合有致，虛實清楚：左虛則右實，虛非全然無力。氣勢要有騰挪；實非全然占煞，精神要貴貫注。緊要全在胸中腰間運化，不在外面。力從人借，氣由脊發，胡能氣由脊發？氣向下沉，由兩肩收入脊骨，注於腰間，此氣之由上而下也，謂之合。由腰形於脊骨，布於兩膊，施於手指，此氣之由下而上也，謂之開。合便是收，開即是放；懂得開合，便知陰陽。到此地位，工用一日，技精一日，漸至從心所欲，罔不如意矣。

Just as you train your Qi to thread through every part of your body, so too must you train your Spirit. Your awareness must reach to every part of your body and even beyond, yet it must also be focused or concentrated. When your Spirit is concentrated your Mind will be able to move the Qi. It is said "Yi Shou Dan Tian" (意守丹田). This means the mind (Yi) is kept on the Dan Tian. The mind will move as you move or do techniques, but it always returns to the abdomen. As you do this you are developing and training your Qi, which is an important part of Spirit. As Qi accumulates it will fill the Dan Tian and the abdomen will be taut like a drum. This is not a rigid tightness. It is the firmness that comes from inflation. Like a drum, Qi has a vibrating and pulsating energy. The Chinese translated here as "agitated" has the sense of motion up and down like a prancing horse or a bubbling well; the word translated here as "smooth" has the sense of smooth motion back and forth. The Spirit of Vitality is an aspect of Shen. It must be lifted up to raise the Spirit as a whole. Shen does not exist in a vacuum. You must develop your techniques, and learn about Yin and Yang. Techniques do not happen by magic—they depend upon a firm grasp of principles, and Jin supported by Qi, all guided by your Spirit. You must understand closing and opening. As you neutralize an attack, you draw your opponent into you, drawing in and borrowing his energy, as well as accumulating the energy of your own body in the Dan Tian. This is called closing, and is done on the inhale. Qi sinks from the shoulders to the Dan Tian down the front of the body. This is Yin and is used to withdraw. At the appropriate time you release the accumulated energy up the spine and out to the hands. This is called opening and is done on the exhale. Qi is raised from the tailbone up the spine to the shoulders and out to the fingers. This is Yang and is used to emit Jin. Again, in all of this, the mind is the master.

Important Training Keys of Stepping and Striking[6-8]

Li, Yi-Yu

Ancient people said: "If (one is) able to lead (the coming force) into the emptiness, (one) can (use) the four ounces to repel one thousand pounds; if (one is) unable to lead (the coming force) into the emptiness, (one) is unable to (use) the four ounces to repel one thousand pounds." This saying is quite correct and conclusive. The beginners are unable to comprehend (this saying), I would like to add a few sentences to explain this. (This will) allow those practitioners who have strong will to learn these techniques (i.e., Taijiquan) be able to follow the opponent and have progress daily.

昔人云，能引進落空，能四兩撥千斤；不能引進落空，不能四兩撥千斤。語甚賅括。初學末由領悟，予加數語以解之；俾有志斯技者，得以從人，庶日進有功矣。

Listening and following are the two first crucial keys of pushing hands. Only if you can listen (i.e., feel) and follow the opponent are you able to adhere and use slight power to lead and neutralize strong force. Though many Taijiquan practitioners know this key, very few are able to really comprehend the profound meaning and are capable of doing it. In the ancient saying, it is stated that the first requirement of reaching this goal is to grasp the trick of leading the opponent's incoming power into emptiness. The author would like to explain this concept again for the sincere Taiji practitioner.

走架打手行功要言 李亦畬

If (you) wish to lead (the coming force) into the emptiness and (use) the four ounces to repel one thousand
pounds, first (you) must know the opponent and
yourself. If (you) wish to know the opponent and yourself, (you) must first give up yourself and follow the
opponent. If (you) wish to give up yourself and follow
(your) opponent, (you) must first gain the advantageous opportunity and situation. If (you) wish to gain
the advantageous opportunity and situation, (you)
must first unite the entire body as a family (i.e., as one
unit). If (you) wish to unite the entire body as a family,
(you) must first have not any faulty place in the entire
body. If (you) wish to have a body without any faulty
place, (you) must first have full Spirit and abundant Qi
filling you like a resonating drum. If (you) wish to have
a full Spirit and abundant Qi, (you) must first raise
up the Spirit of Vitality and the Spirit not dispersed
externally. If (you) wish to keep the Spirit from disper-
sion externally, (you) must first condense the Spirit
and Qi to the bone marrow. If (you) wish to condense
the Spirit and Qi to the bone marrow, (you) must first
have strength on the front sides of your thighs, your
two shoulders are loose and opening, and the Qi is
sunk downward.

欲要引進落空，四兩撥千斤，先要知己知彼。欲要
知己知彼，先要舍己從人。欲要舍己從人，先要得
機得勢。欲要得機得勢，先要周身一家。欲要周身
一家，先要周身無有缺陷。欲要周身無有缺陷，先
要神氣鼓蕩。欲要神氣鼓蕩，先要提起精神，神不
外散。欲要神不外散，先要神氣收斂入骨。欲要神
氣收斂入骨，先要兩股前節有力、兩肩鬆開、氣向
下沉。

The author believes that in order to use a slight force to lead
strong incoming force into emptiness, you must first build up your
sensitivity and receptiveness (i.e., Listening Jin). Feeling is a language
that builds up the communication between you and your opponent.

If you have high sensitivity, you can know your opponent. Only if you can know your opponent's intention and your capability of fighting have you built up the foundation of leading the opponent's force into emptiness.

However, before you can know your opponent, you must also know the trick of following Jin. Following Jin means the yielding which allows your opponent's force to enter, but only under your control. If you are unable to yield and allow the incoming force to enter, you will be resisting, and will generate double-weighting (i.e., mutual resistance). In this case, your use of force against force will prevent you from neutralizing the incoming force. From following the opponent, you start to understand the opponent. Only if you can understand the opponent can you control the entire situation and gain advantageous timing and winning conditions.

But the trick to gaining the advantageous situation is not an easy task. In order to gain the advantageous situation, you must first learn how to unite and activate your body as one unit. If your body cannot act as an integrated whole, top to bottom and left to right, you will create a faulty place (i.e., create an opportunity) for your opponent's attack.

In order to move the body with a high level of harmonious coordination, you must have strong and abundant Qi and a high Spirit of alertness (i.e., high sensitivity). In order to reach this goal, you must first raise up the Spirit of Vitality and learn to condense the Spirit (i.e., concentrate). Once you can do so, you will be able to use the concentrated mind to condense the Qi (i.e., to store) the Qi at the bone marrow for further emission. Storing the Qi at the bone marrow is Yin (i.e., bone marrow breathing) and emitting the Jin is Yang (i.e., skin breathing) which manifests the Jin into external form. In order to have a condensed Spirit and Qi, you must first examine your postures. The legs are strong and firm to build up a solid root. Without this solid root, your body will not be centered and balanced. Furthermore, you must always remember to keep the arms loose (i.e., drop elbows and sink shoulders) and keep the Qi down in the Lower Dan Tian. Whenever the Qi is dispersed from the Lower Dan Tian, the mind is scattered and the Spirit will not be condensed.

From this paragraph, you can see that the first concern for reaching the crucial skill of using four ounces to repel one thousand pounds is learning how to regulate your body. Only if your body is centered and rooted can you have a relaxed and balanced physical body. Next, you should regulate your mind (i.e., Spirit). With high Spirit and coordination of correct breathing, your Spirit can be raised up to a highly sensitive level. When this happens, you will be very alert in responding to incoming force. That means you have established a high level of Listening Jin. With this high level of Listening Jin, you can use four ounces to repel one thousand pounds.

Jins originate from the bottom of feet, exchange in the legs, fill and store in the chest, manifest on the shoulders, are mastered from the waist, and coordinate through the two arms on the top corresponding to the two legs below. Jin changes internally, withdraw is close and release is opening. When calm, all calm. Calmness is close, and hidden within closing is opening. When move, all move. Movement is opening, and hidden within opening is closing. When touches, (the entire body) then turning and coiling automatically. Must without using (any) force, then can lead (the coming force) into emptiness and (use) the four ounces to repel one thousand pounds.

勁起于腳跟，變換在腿，含蓄在胸，運動在兩肩，
主宰在腰，上于兩膊相系，下于兩腿相隨。勁由內
換，收便是合，放即是開，靜則俱靜。靜是合，合
中寓開。動則俱動，動是開，開中有合，觸之則旋
轉自如。無不得力，才能引進落空，四兩撥千斤。

For Jins originating from the bottom of the feet, you will be rooted when Jins are emitted. If there is a forward, there is a backward. The backward is Yin, and provides the force for forward emitting, which is Yang. Once you have grasped the trick of Yin and Yang balance, you have comprehended a crucial key to Jin's manifestation. Since the Jins originate from the legs, it is the legs that can vary the strategy of every movement. The chest is a bow that can store the Jin (i.e., Peng Jin). When the Jin manifests in the arms, the shoulders are the key to connecting them to the body. When this connection is adequate, the Jin can be manifested from the arms skillfully and efficiently. However, the waist still controls the Jin so generated. The waist directs and governs the Jin to the desired direction. In order to manifest the Jin, connection areas such as the shoulders and hip joints make the entire body one unit.

Yet the origin of the Jin is still internal. It is generated from the Yi, and from the Yi the Qi is led and power is generated. When the mind and the posture are withdrawing, it is not just for yielding and neutralizing. Instead, it is also storing Jin and preparing for its emission. Once you have emitted, you immediately think of withdrawing. Withdrawing is Yin, which stores the Jin, and emitting is Yang, which manifests the Jin. Therefore, closing of the postures is the beginning of opening and opening is the beginning of closing. Yin and Yang are mutually linked together and cannot be separated. Once you can exchange the Yin (i.e., insubstantial) and Yang (i.e., substantial), any slight touch from your opponent can be neutralized without force. Then you have grasped the trick of using four ounces to repel one thousand pounds.

Normally, (when you are) stepping and posturing (i.e., practicing), (it) is a Gongfu of knowing yourself. Once moving, first ask yourself if the above criteria are matched. (Even if) it is slightly unmatched, change immediately. Therefore, when stepping and posturing (i.e., practicing), (you) must be slow instead of fast. (However) when (you are) striking hands (i.e., fighting), (it) is the Gongfu of knowing the opponent. Though moving or still decided from knowing opponent, (I) still ask myself. (If) I arrange good (i.e., ready), when the opponent touches me, I do not move (him even) slightly. (I) take the opportunity and enter to intercept and adhere the coming moving. The opponent will naturally bounce out. If there is any urgent place within yourself, then it is (because) not able to solve the problem of double-weighting. (In this case, you) must find the solution within the keys of Yin-Yang and opening-closing. That is what is said: "Knowing the opponent, knowing yourself, hundred battles, hundred victories.

平日走架，是知己功夫，一動勢先問自己周身合上
數項合否？稍有不合，即速改換，所以走架要慢不
要快。打手是知人功夫，動靜固是知人，仍是問己
。自己安排得好，人一挨我，我不動，彼絲毫趁勢
而入，接定彼勁，彼自跌出。如自己有不得力處，
便是雙重未化，要于陰陽開合中求之。所謂知己知
彼，百戰百勝也。

When you train by yourself, it is the Gongfu of self-refinement and self-perfection. Therefore, when you practice by yourself, you should always keep the above training criteria in your mind. You should not allow any mistake, and always shoot for deeper understanding and potential neutralization. In order to reach this goal, you must first train yourself slowly. When you are slow, your mind will be calm. When your mind is calm, your feelings and thought will be deep and profound. This will lead you to a deeper comprehension. Deep and profound comprehension is the key to refining your practice.

However, when you train with a partner, the character of your practice will be different from solo practice. Instead, there is an exchange of techniques and Qi between you and your opponent. While calmly moving, you must not only know yourself but also know your opponent. Nevertheless, your mind is still defensive. You still ask yourself if you are following the opponent or you are resisting the opponent. If you can feel (i.e., listen), follow (i.e., yield), and adhere skillfully, you will be able to lead (i.e., neutralize) the incoming force with a slight force. When this happens, you can not only lead the incoming force into emptiness, but you can also uproot your opponent and make him lose balance and fall. If you continue to feel awkward in applying the above key skills, then you are still bound in the knot of mutual resistance (i.e., double weighting), perhaps without even being conscious of it. It also means that you have not yet really comprehended the essence of Yin and Yang (i.e., closing and opening). You must practice until you can comprehend the meaning of this and can execute these skills efficiently. When you can, you have reached the level of knowing yourself and your opponent, and have already won all of your battles.

Song of Taijiquan Applications[13]

Li, Yi-Yu

太極拳體用歌 李亦畬

Marvelous Taijiquan, (its) transportation methods (i.e., techniques) pattern nature. Soft as jade ring, (stay) with Taiji illustration always. The entire body (acts) as one Qi, top and bottom without leaning and deviation. Stepping is like a cat's walking, transport the Qi as the spiraling (i.e., coiling) of silk. Once move, nothing without moving, once calm all calm. On the top, the head must be suspended, at the bottom, sink the Qi to the (Lower) Dan Tian. Drop the shoulders and sink the elbows, arc the back and contain the chest. The tailbone is upright naturally, the body is loosened and the Qi is abundant and full.

妙哉太極拳，運行法自然。綿綿如玉環，
著著太極圖。渾身如一氣，上下無斜偏。
邁步如貓行，運氣把絲盤。一動無不動，
一靜俱寂然。上要頂頭懸，下氣沉丹田。
垂肩與墜肘，拔背把胸含。尾閭自中正，
體鬆氣騰然。

The art of Taijiquan is marvelous because all its theory and applications follow the natural pattern of the Dao. It is as soft as Jade Ring (also called Huang Ting, 黃庭 or Zhong Ting, 中庭). According to Chinese Daoist Qigong,
Jade Ring means the central area (i.e., Yu Huan Xue, 玉環穴) in the abdomen, where the Spiritual fetus resides. This place
is completely soft and natural, which allows the Qi to accumulate and the Spiritual fetus to grow. All of the derivations of Taiji theory and its applications all follow the Yin and Yang principle. This is the most basic concept in Taijiquan.

Since Taijiquan is an internal art, more than just learning the external postures, you must also train to fill up the Lower Dan Tian with a sustained abundance of Qi, and to use the mind to lead the Qi so you can manifest it into physical form. In addition, in order to have a firm root, you must first learn to be balanced, and then you can center yourself. The body must be upright yet relaxed. When you step, it is as light and agile as a cat. When you transport the Qi, it is as slender, soft, and natural as silk. Once moved, the entire body moves as one unit and once it is calm, the entire body is calm as a mountain. On the top of your body, your head feels suspended upward to raise up the Spirit of Vitality, while your Qi deeply sinks to the Lower Dan Tian. The downward Qi's sinking is Yin, and the manifestation of Spirit is Yang. When the Qi sinks deeply, the Spirit's uprising is powerful.

In order to have a firm root to manifest the Jin, the elbows and the shoulders must be dropped. This will provide you with a firm connection of the arm to the body for Jin's manifestation. In addition, when the elbows and shoulders are sinking, you are also sealing the vital area under the armpit from your opponent's attack. The first key posture of Taijiquan is Peng (wardoff). In order to execute this posture correctly, you should settle your chest inward while arcing your back. When you are doing so, you have already created a first posture either for offense or defense. The upright tailbone implies the torso being held upward, though the entire body is relaxed. When the body is relaxed, the Qi can circulate smoothly and freely.

Use the Yi and not the Li, turning the waist to turn over (i.e., control) the body. The root (of the Jin) is on the feet and growing upward, understanding (the usage of) legs and waist carefully and profoundly. Jin is emitted from the spine, (it) reaches (through) arm to the fingers. Extend the tendons and pull the bone, settle down the waist to manifest on the fingertips. (When) the fingers feel slightly swelling, (it implies) the Qi arrives and is manifested in the physical body. All of these are (originated) from Xin (i.e., emotional mind) and Yi (i.e., wisdom mind), do not treat it as the clumsy force. Insubstantial and substantial must be discriminated clearly, soft and hard exchange following the situation. Yin and Yang must mutually support each other, to and fro must have an exchange.

用意不用力，轉腰把身翻。根在腳上升，
腿腰認的端。勁由脊中發，膀臂到指尖。
伸筋與拔骨，坐腕展指端。手指覺微漲，
氣到體自顯。此全是心意，莫當拙力言。
虛實分清楚，剛柔隨變遷。陰陽要相濟，
往返須轉變。

In order to lead the Qi, you must learn how to use your Yi instead of muscular force, which can make you tense. The Jin is generated from the feet, steered by the waist and manifested at the hands. Therefore, the waist is the major key to controlling the body's action. Jin is stored in the chest and the spine (i.e., bow of torso) and therefore it is emitted from the torso. Once the Jin is emitted, it reaches to the fingertips through the arms. If you are not using muscular force (i.e., Li), your Jin will be soft as a whip. When this happens, the tendons in the joints will be extended and pulled. Once the Jin reaches the fingers, settle down your wrist. This will allow you to manifest Jin efficiently and powerfully. In order to unify the internal Jin (i.e., Nei Jin) and external Jin (i.e., Wai Jin), you must learn how to use the Yi to lead the Qi to the fingers. When this happens, you will feel the sensation of swelling in the fingers. All of this is generated from the Xin (i.e., emotional mind) and Yi (i.e., wisdom mind). While the Xin can raise up the Spirit of fighting, the Yi is still needed to control the Xin. This is internal and not an external muscular power manifestation.

When you apply the Jin, insubstantial and substantial must be clearly distinguished. If you are skillful in Jin, you should be able to manifest the Jin as hard or soft as you wish depending on the situation. This means Yin and Yang mutually support each other and can exchange with each other.

Qi is full and agitated following the situations (or postures), the Spirit must be condensed internally. Movements are arisen from the calmness, though moving, the calmness is still within. The Spirit leads and the Qi follows, (when) the waist moves, the palm and the wrist are connected. The stepping follows the variation of the situations (or postures), the hands and eyes are the first to encounter. Fast and slow follow the movement of the opponent, simply the posture of sinking should not be postponed (i.e., ignored). Do not lose and do not resist, every posture must lead first. After leading the (coming Jin) into the emptiness, emitting Jin as the water from a bubbling well. It does not matter if he is a steel metal fellow, (use) the four ounces to repel one thousand pounds.

氣隨勢鼓蕩，神要內中斂。動從靜中升，
雖動靜猶然。神領氣隨到，腰動掌腕連。
步隨勢變化，手眼照當前。快慢隨人動，
單沉勢勿延。不丟與不頂，勢勢要領先。
引進落空後，發勁似湧泉。任他金鋼漢，
四兩撥千金。

When you apply the Taijiquan techniques, the Yi should lead the Qi smoothly and strongly. Moreover, in order to avoid confusion and emotional disturbance, the Spirit should be condensed. When the Spirit is condensed, the mind will be calm. It is from the calmness that judgment is accurate and clear. Therefore, even if you are in a serious combat situation, the mind should continue to be calmed through condensing the Spirit. When the Spirit is arisen, the Qi can be led efficiently and effectively. When the Qi is led from the Lower Dan Tian (waist area) to the arms and palms, it is connected as one single unit. The stepping always follows the techniques and the strategies. Keep the eyes alert, reflect the situation to the brain quickly, and react in the hands immediately.

Do not move randomly but follow the opponent's speed. When the opponent is slow, I am also slow. When the opponent is fast, I also move fast. Only then can I listen, follow, and adhere with the opponent. During pushing hands, sinking is the key to destroying the opponent's intention of attacking. If you can sink the opponent's force downward at all times, you can put him in a defensive situation. Once you can put your opponent into a defensive profile, if you are also able to stick and adhere with him, you will control the entire situation. When this happens, you can lead the opponent's attack into emptiness and immediately emit your Jin easily and successfully. If you have reached this level, even if you face a strong tough opponent, you are still able to repel one thousand pounds with only four ounces.

Song of Thirteen Postures[1,8,12]

Li, Yi-Yu

十三勢歌 李亦畬

The secret of thirteen total postures, few people have learned since ancient times. (Those) who have the predestined relationship (with me) have a deep fortune (today), (I) break the rules and tell you (this secret). Arc the arms must be round and alive (i.e., Peng Jin), (when) the hands go out (i.e., contact with opponent), (first) ask the feeling (i.e., Ting Jin). When the opponent('s power) is void I press (i.e., Ji Jin) and when the opponent('s power) is solid, (I) sink (my) elbow and repel (i.e., Hua Jin). Wardoff diagonally (i.e., Lie Jin) upward from outside, (the opponent) will lean backward and cannot stand firmly.

> 十三總勢訣，自古少人學。有緣深造化，
> 破格為君說。繃臂要圓活，出手問知覺。
> 敵空使我擠，敵實墜肘撥。由外斜掤上，
> 後仰站不著。

Though many Taijiquan practitioners have understood that Taijiquan was founded on the basic thirteen postures, still, only few people ever really comprehend the secret of its essence. The author in this article would like to reveal these secrets to those people who read this article (i.e., predestined relationship).

The first crucial key to apply the thirteen postures is arcing the arms and to form a discovered circle right in front of the chest. This implies Peng Jin (i.e., wardoff). You must also know how to keep this Jin alive and skillful. Once in contact with the opponent, pay careful, soft, and concentrated attention to the feeling of touch (i.e., Listening Jin). The feeling is the language of mutual communication between you and your opponent. If you are very sensitive and skillful in this feeling, you can grasp the opponent's intention. From listening, if the opponent has a void, use the Ji Jin (i.e., Press Jin) to force him to lose his balance. However, if the opponent's force is solid and strong, sink the elbow to build up a firm neutralization foundation, and lead and repel the opponent's power downward (i.e., Neutralization Jin). After the neutralization, immediately use the Lie Jin (i.e., Split Jin) to bounce the opponent off balance.

After Lu (i.e, rollback), An (i.e, push), and Peng (i.e., wardoff), sink the shoulder and turn the muscles/tendons on the waist. Keep rollback and follow the opponent to neutralize (the coming force), trick the opponent into the empty (i.e., exposed) cavity. Press (i.e., Ji Jin) is frequently used on the side, sinking down to shock the opponent. (From) turning movement to strike forward, (when it is) far to gauge the ground is flat or not. Within the push (i.e., An Jin) must include closing, first downward and then return (the force). Turning upward and then push forward, defeat the opponent ten feet away. Pluck (i.e., Cai Jin) must use the solid force, (if the force is) too light, it is not effective. First sink down from the top, pluck sideways horizontally passing (your) body. Split (Lie) attacks by turning horizontally, quick knife (hand) to cut (attack) the face and neck. (If) the opponent is urgently close to strike me, split hands (i.e., Lie Jin) is the first technique to be used (to solve the problem).

擾按繃臂後，沉肩轉腰肋。擾著隨化走，
誘敵入空穴。擠多偏摸用，下沉敵驚愕。
轉動向前打，遠側地平坡。按中要帶合，
先下後回折。上轉再前按，丈外把敵挫。
採必用實力，過輕無效果。從上先沉下，
平採身旁過。挒打平旋轉，快刀斬額脖。
迫進來打我，挒手為先著。

After you have applied the technique of Lu (i.e., rollback), An (i.e., push), or Peng (i.e., wardoff), your opponent will be in an imbalanced or confused situation. Therefore, you should immediately sink your elbows and shoulders, and use your waist to turn the body. This will allow you to generate sideways power to bounce him off balance. After neutralization, continue to use Lu to lead the opponent into emptiness and expose his vital area for your attack. When you use Ji (i.e., press), often the force should be sideways diagonally. If you simply press forward, it is easier for your opponent to retreat by stepping backward and escape. However, if you press sideways slightly, you will make your opponent lose his balance easily. In order to generate a firm press, you must first sink and build down a firm root for yourself. Only then, can the pressing power be strong and surprise the opponent.

When you strike forward, the power is directed from the waist's turning. If the opponent is far away, you must be careful if the ground is flat or not when you step forward. If you use An (i.e., push), it is important that the An power is closed instead of opened. When the An Jin is closed, it is solid and strong, and when the An Jin is opened, it can be neutralized by the opponent easily. First push downward and this will cause your opponent's resistance. When this happens, immediately change the strategy and return your An force and this will make the opponent's effort of resistance in vain. Immediately after returning, lead the incoming force upward and then push forward again. This will neutralize the resisting force and lead the opponent up and off his root. When this happens, immediately push forward to bounce him off balance.

When you use Cai (i.e., pluck), the force must be solid. That means you must continue your Cai Jin until the opponent loses his balance. If the Cai Jin is too light, the opponent will regain his balance quickly and your effort will be in vain. When Cai is used, first pluck the opponent's arm downward and to the side of your body. This will take your opponent off balance.

When you use Lie (i.e., split), the force is from sideways. This force can be used to attack the opponent's neck or head. This sideways force can also make the opponent fall. If the opponent is urgently close to me, Lie is the first technique to use.

Use Zhou (i.e., elbow) when (the opponent) is near, bend the arm and aim the chest tendons. If the opponent presses my elbows, blossom the flowers (and the opponent) cannot evade to any place. (When using) the bump (i.e., Kao), first search for the triangular, poke the groin and the eyes are looking downward and sideways. The waist and the body are turning at the same time, (you will) send him (i.e., the opponent) to see the Yan Lo (i.e., king of the hell). (When) stepping forward, (you should) occupy the central palace (i.e., center door), the urgent pressure (generated) is hard for (your) opponent to endure. When the opponent is close (range), step only half step, (this will) avoid the opportunity used by the opponent. (When) stepping backward (i.e., retreat), (the retreating stepping) must be rubbing one after another (i.e., tight stepping), (if the opponent) is looking for the gap, there is no trace and shadow. Gu (i.e., beware of the left) is used with three is on the front (i.e., 30% of the weight is on the front leg), Pan (i.e., look to the right) is used with seven on the rear (i.e., 70% weight on the rear leg). Tu (i.e., central equilibrium) does not leave the position, contain the chest and loosen the waist. Profoundly comprehend the thirteen postures, every posture is unlimited marvelous.

肘在近處使，屈臂指胸肋。敵若按我肘，
開花無處躲。靠先找三角，插襠眼下斜。
腰身一齊轉，送他見閻羅。進步搶中宮，
逼勢人難容。相近上半步，免被敵人乘。
退步先後擦，尋隙無蹤影。顧在三前使，
盼在七星用。中土不離位，含胸把腰鬆。
細體十三勢，勢勢妙無窮。

When the opponent is in close range, attack and defend with the elbows instead of the hands. Generally speaking, the power generated from the elbow is much stronger than that of the hands. Furthermore, in short range, the elbow can be fast and a surprise to the opponent. If you use the elbow to strike, aim for the tendons on the ribs, sharply. This will cause the muscles around his lungs to contract and consequently seal the breath. If the opponent uses An (i.e., push downward) to neutralize the elbow attack, immediately use the fist to attack his face, like the blossoming of a flower.

When you use Kao (i.e., bump), the angle of approaching the opponent is very important. If you can catch the correct angle and enter the space between the opponent's legs, you will occupy the empty door for you to enter. This angle will allow you to attack his groin and also to bounce him off balance easily. When you change your angle for the Kao attack, you must turn your body as well to avoid your opponent's attack to your exposed areas. In addition, if you can turn the body with the proper angling, you can line up your body into a good posture to execute strong techniques. According to Buddhists, Yan Lo (閻羅王) is the King who is in charge of hell.

Central palace (i.e., Zhong Gong, 中宮) means the area between the legs. If your opponent's right leg is forward, the central palace is on his left side. If you step in this central palace from the opponent's left hand side, it is entering the "empty door" (Kong Men, 空門). Therefore, when you step forward (i.e., Qian Jin), you are always trying to enter this central palace. This will put your opponent in an urgent and dangerous situation, because the front side of his body will be exposed to your attack. However, do not step in too deeply. This may put you into a dangerous situation. Half a step is adequate.

When you step back (i.e., Hou Tui), keep your legs closed and do not open wide. This would allow your opponent to attack you. If you step backward carefully with your legs closed, you will be more firm and rooted.

When you lead the force to your left (i.e., beware of the left, Zuo Gu), you should apply it only if 30% or less of your weight is on your front leg. If you have too much weight on the front leg and try to use power to your left, you will be leaning forward, and can be led and neutralized easily. However, if you intend to apply the power to your right, keep 70% of your weight on your rear leg. Eventually, this implies that when you use your force either to your left or to your right, do not place too much weight on your front leg. You can be led and leaned forward, and lose your balance.

However, no matter which postures you apply, you should always keep physically and mentally centered. According to the five elements theory, the central equilibrium belongs to the earth. The key to keeping this center is arcing your back and chest (i.e., Peng Jin), and keeping your waist area loose and soft. When the waist is soft, your opponent will not be able to find your root and uproot you.

Secret of Eight Words[13]

Li, Yi-Yu

八
字
歌

李亦畬

Peng (i.e., wardoff) arms manifested diagonally as the crescent moon, bend the front knee slightly and the rear palms are round. How much weight (i.e., force or potential) the opponent has, (when) the Peng arms touch to gauge (the weight) as scale. (When) the opponent's Jin emitted (against me), I seal and pluck, (when) the opponent('s postures) as hollow, I use Ji (i.e., press). The top to the bottom, one group of Qi, (it is) like long python occupies the ground.

> 掤臂斜出月上弦，前膝微拱後掌圓。
> 對方斤兩有多少，掤臂觸之似稱盤。
> 敵勁出頭我封采，對方凹陷我擠然。
> 上下渾身一團氣，猶如長蛇撲地盤。

When Peng Jin is manifested, both arms are arced as the crescent moon. This will allow you to yield and lead the opponent's oncoming Jin into position for your further neutralization. When you use Peng Jin to yield, you should not keep both of your arms horizontal, because that will allow your opponent to find the counter to your Peng Jin. However, if you manifest your Peng Jin diagonally, then your opponent will lose balance and centering. When you execute Peng Jin, not only are the arms round, but also the palms are round and the knees are bent so you sink down firmly, very deeply. When the palms are round, they are not stiff but soft, and when the knees squat down, the root can be firm.

In pushing hands, Peng Jin is commonly used to measure the strength of an opponent's power and gauge his skill. From Peng Jin, you can flow to other Jins easily. If the incoming force is strong, simply yield and neutralize, and follow with a seal or pluck. However, if I feel the opponent's force is weak and there is a gap to enter, immediately,

I use Ji (i.e., press) to force him off balance. All of these applications and manifestation rely on internal Yi and Qi. If you are so confident, you will be like a python controlling its territory.

(Move) hands as the deer turning its head, the palm is high and the arm is low, postures are freely (moved). The Spirit and the Yi are manifested completely on the palms, the waist and the legs are (moving) coordinated as the (floating) boat following the stream. Stick and adhere do not leave the central earth, the reason is within the Lu (i.e., rollback) there is leading. (If) there is Lu (i.e., rollback) without (following) with Ji (i.e, press), the Lu is useless. (However, if) there is Ji without Lu, then the Ji will also be in vain.

手法好似鹿回頭，掌高手低勢自由。
神意全在掌中現，腰腿一致順水舟。
沾粘不離中土位，攦中帶引是根由。
有攦無擠空自攦，無攦有擠枉出頭。

This paragraph is talking about Lu. When you apply the Lu technique, the arms are like two antlers of the deer and the turning is powerful yet delicate as a deer's turning of its head. When you apply Lu, the hands are high and the elbows are low. However, do not be restricted in a definitive posture. You should be able to move and change freely. The Spirit must be high and the Yi leading the Qi should be strong and manifested on the palms. This means that the sense of enemy must be strong so you can be alert. When you apply the Lu technique, the root and the coordination of the waist are the most important factors. Without the firm root and the governing of the Lu Jin, your neutralization will not be effective.

Stick and adhere with the opponent's arm while keeping yourself firmly centered and deeply rooted. This is because there is leading Jin within Lu Jin. Lu Jin is generally built by three Jins: Yielding Jin, Leading Jin, and Neutralizing Jin. When you lead the opponent's power into emptiness, you must first have a firm root and mobile, alive waist movements.

However, Lu Jin is normally used together with Ji Jin (i.e., press). Often, when you apply Lu Jin, you will neutralize the oncoming force and put the opponent into an awkward and unbalanced situation. At this moment, if you apply Ji Jin immediately, you will be able to catch the opportunity to change defense into offense. Similarly, if you apply Ji Jin without first neutralizing your opponent's incoming, your Ji will not be effective since your opponent is not in a disadvantageous situation.

(When) the technique of press (Ji) is emitted, (it) is better than arcing bridge (Gong Qiao). In the diagonal, there is a closed contact is (the way) of making the Qi abundant. When encountering An (i.e., push), Da (i.e., striking), and Ji (i.e., press), first rollback and neutralize. (In order to) lead (the coming force) to enter the emptiness, (you must) search for (i.e., pay attention to) the single arm. Keep the arcing bridge closed on the opponent's arms. First sink down and then forward without encircling (i.e., hesitating). After press and then rollback, (coming force) cannot be lead and enter (the emptiness). After rollback without press, (the effort) is empty.

擠手打出賽拱橋，斜中帶摸竟氣豪。
逢按打擠先履化，引進落空單臂找。
拱橋閉著敵膀臂，先沉後前勢無繞。
擠又從攦無引進，攦後無擠是空著。

This paragraph is talking about Ji Jin. Gong Qiao (拱橋) means arcing bridge in Chinese martial arts society. This means the opponent's hands are bridging together and exchanging techniques. In Taijiquan, it is commonly called pushing hands. Normally, when you are in a pushing hands situation, both you and your opponent balance each other. However, whenever you have a chance, you should step in and apply Ji. When you apply Ji, the direction of Ji should be from the opponent's side. If you apply it from the front, your opponent has a firm root, and the Ji Jin will not be effective. Moreover, since Ji Jin is only effective at the close range, you must stick and adhere with your opponent closely, keeping the Qi abundant.

Lu and Ji are frequently used together. When you encounter An, Da, or Ji, you should first use Lu to neutralize the coming offensive force and then immediately apply the Ji Jin. However, when you apply Lu, you should only stay on one side of your opponent's body (i.e., single arm). This will allow you to apply the Ji from the side. Therefore, the entire strategy against the incoming three techniques is to first sink the force downward and sideways (i.e., Lu) and then use Ji without hesitation. You should remember that usually, Ji is applied right after Lu—the order should not be reversed—and both are always applied together.

Da (i.e., strike) and An (i.e., push) are as the tiger pouncing on the lamb. The waist, legs, and arms must be properly (situated) individually. First sink down, next bring back and then emit An (i.e., push). Surely, (you) will throw the opponent away at the place. (When you apply) An (i.e., push), Peng (i.e., wardoff), Lu (i.e., rollback), and Hua (i.e., neutralize), (you) must be very careful. The elbow does not pass the (front) knee though slightly (over) is no problem. (When) the opponent steps back and uses Cai (i.e., pluck) on me, (I) step forward and use Zhou (i.e., elbow) and Kao (i.e, bump) to injure the opponent.

打按好似虎撲羊，腰腿手臂各相當。
先沉後帶再按出，定將敵人擲當場。
按掤攦化須注意，肘不過膝略無妨。
對方撤步來採我，進步肘靠將敵傷。

This paragraph is talking about attacking by An or Da. When you emit these two Jins, they must be as powerful and aggressive as a tiger pouncing on his prey. The Jin originates from the legs, is directed by the waist, and manifests at the arms. In order to manifest Jin powerfully and act as one single unit (i.e., soft whip), the coordination of the legs, waist, and arms is the most important element. If there is any slightly improper coordination, the power emitted will be weakened.

When you apply An, first you should sink the incoming force downward and backward to yield and neutralize. This will create an advantageous situation for your An and Da. If you apply this properly, you will be able to defeat your opponent easily.

When you use the An, Peng, Lu, and Hua Jins, you should pay attention to an important alignment. That is, your elbows should not go past the front knee. Still, as long as you keep yourself firmly centered and deeply rooted, there is no problem if your elbow passes over the front knee only just slightly. When you apply the An and Da Jin, if your opponent uses Cai (i.e., pluck) to neutralize your attack with retreating steps, you should immediately take the opportunity to step forward and use either elbow to attack, or your body (e.g., shoulder or hip) to bump him off balance.

Cai (i.e., pluck) is like an ape monkey picks up the immortal peach. Sink downward and bring (the coming force) diagonally (i.e., sideways and downward) to attract the opponent to attack. (When) stepping backward to Cai (i.e., pluck) the wrist, must old and hot (i.e., skillful and aggressive). (If the opponent does) not lean and break (the root), (the effort) is in vain. It does not matter (if the opponent) uses the Peng (i.e., wardoff), An (i.e., push), Quan (i.e., fist strike), or Zhang (i.e., palm strike), when encountering the application of pluck, (the coming techniques) dissolved as ice. (When) using pluck, (you) must carefully prevent the opponent's Zhou (i.e., elbow) and Kao (i.e., bump).

(If you are able) to keep the central palace (i.e., central equilibrium), (you are) able to throw (the opponent) away as wish.

採似猿猴摘仙桃，沉後斜帶引敵偷。
退步採腕要老辣，不傾不脆枉徒勞。
無論掤按與拳掌，採用遇之似冰消。
用採切防敵肘靠，守著中宮任意拋。

This paragraph is talking about Cai. According to Chinese legend, if you eat of the peaches grown in the heavenly kingdom, you can become immortal. When you apply Cai, you should not grab and be tensed. It is like an ape stealing an immortal peach in the heavens; be quiet, quick, and soft. First, after you have plucked the opponent's arm (i.e., normally at the wrists, elbows, or shoulders), sink the power downward and bring the opponent to your side. When this happens, your opponent will have a chance to use his elbow or shoulder to attack you. Therefore, when you apply the Cai, the power must be solid and aggressive until your opponent loses his root and balance. This will prevent him from attacking you.

Cai is specially designed to work against Peng, An, Quan, and Palm Jins. If you can apply Cai correctly, you can lead the incoming attacks into emptiness (i.e., dissolved as ice). The only thing you must be aware of is that when you apply Cai Jin, you must keep yourself centered and balanced (i.e., central equilibrium). If you do not have this strong root and center, you will not be able to handle the incoming elbow attack and bumping (e.g., shoulder stroke).

(When) Lie (i.e., split) strike with sideways power (Heng Jin), (it is) emitted with surprise and springing (force). Dodge away from central door and walk with spiral (path). Single hand to sweep the opponent's neck and head horizontally. (The speed) is like a speedy horse to urge the windmill turning. (If opponent applies) Lie (i.e., split) strike (to me), (I) still need to use the Lie (i.e., split) strike to dissolve (the coming Lie). (When) opponent treats me politely, I return with polite (i.e., same way). The shoulders are turning following the waist (as) a dragon is turning its body. Do remember do not hesitate and be clumsy and lose the natural (i.e., naturally and skillfully).

捯打橫勁出驚彈，避開中門走螺旋。
單手平掃適頸頂，予似快馬摧磨轉。
捯手還須捯手破，彼以禮來我禮還。
肩隨腰轉龍轉身，切忌遲呆不天然。

This paragraph is talking about Lie. Lie Jin is commonly applied with sideward force (i.e., Heng Jin). When Lie Jin is used, if your opponent knows your intention, it will not work effectively. Therefore, you must attack with surprise and with bouncing force. When you attack, you approach the opponent sideways (i.e., avoiding the central door). This will allow you to attack the opponent's neck or head with a sideways horizontal hand strike. The key to making this technique successful is speed. This technique can be detected by the opponent easily. If you are slow, your opponent will have a good chance to retreat or neutralize your attack.

Lie is commonly used against Lie. When you apply Lie, you are using the entire body's force to split or to rend the opponent. Therefore, the force should be strong and the entire body rooted and completely controlled by the waist. When you apply Lie, you cannot hesitate and be clumsy. This will allow your opponent to sense your intention and your attack will be useless.

(When using) Zhou (i.e., elbow) to strike, (it) is as a cow bowing its head. Blossom the flowers (with) linking attack as (you) wish. This (technique) is used with closed range when Cai (i.e., pluck) is applied (on you). (If it is) used at the long range, (you will) earn the shame by the opponent. (When) the opponent uses Cai (i.e., pluck) to seal me, (I) apply (elbow stroke) following the (opponent's) posture. Pointing the elbow to the ribs' tendons, (the opponent's) life will be rested (i.e, ended). (When) using the elbow (to strike), the most fearful (technique) against (you) is the posture of playing guitar. When encountered, turn the body (to protect) my throat.

肘打好似牛低頭，開花連環任自由。
此是近取一採手，遠距用之氣人羞。
對方封采隨勢用，肘指肋脅一命休。
用肘最怕琵琶勢，遇之轉身我咽喉。

When you apply Zhou either for defense or offense, your neck and head area will be opened for a strike. Therefore, in such a short range, you must protect your neck and head by bowing and hiding the head behind the posture. If Zhou has been neutralized, immediately use your fist to strike the opponent's face continuously. Zhou can only be used for a short range situation. If you do not understand this principle and apply it without the proper range, you will be laughed at by your opponent (i.e., the technique is in vain).

Normally, Zhou is used against Cai. When your opponent uses Cai on you, simply reposition yourself, follow the opponent's Cai force and use the elbow to attack him. The best place for your elbow's attack is the rib area, which can cause the muscles around the lungs to contract and therefore seal the breath. However, when you apply Zhou, you must be very careful. If your opponent uses both of his hands to lock your shoulder and elbow (i.e., playing guitar), he will be able to neutralize your elbow attack and follow with an attack to your head and throat. Once you have sensed his intention to apply play guitar on you, immediately turn your head and retreat quickly to avoid the attack.

(When) stepping forward to use Kao (i.e., bump) strike, it is as competing with the swimming dragon. (When) Kao is used, the leg straightly (i.e., directly) enters the opponent's crotch. (When striking) from the bottom to the top, turn the body urgently. (Use) the shoulder to strike the opponent's chest, do not show mercy.

Absolutely do not (use) single leg to support the body (i.e., center), which allows the opponent the space to withdraw. Kao strike is frequently varied from the Cai. (When) the opponent dodges (my bump), I use pluck to accomplish my technique.

進步打靠賽游龍，靠腿直入敵襠中。
由下斜上急轉身，肩打敵胸不容情。
切忌一腿不鼎主，致使對方有餘容。
靠打多由採手變，敵閃我採招法成。

When you use Kao to attack, you must be as swift as a swimming dragon so you can close in and enter the opponent's body space, from long range to short range. The angle of entering is between the opponent's legs (i.e., crotch). This will put the opponent in a disadvantageous position. In order to bump the opponent off balance and uproot him, the bumping force must go from low to high. Once you have a chance to use the shoulder to stroke the opponent, you should act quickly and show no mercy. This is simply because in such a short range situation, if you show mercy, you have provided a good chance for your opponent's counter-attack. When you bump the opponent off balance, the easy mistake is to lean on one leg (i.e., place most of the weight on one leg). If you do so, you will have lost your center. Once your opponent uses Cai against you, you will have a serious problem. Like Cai and Zhou, Cai and Kao are often used together.

Song of Transporting and Applying Spirit and Qi[13]

Li, Yi-Yu

神氣運行歌 李亦畬

Qi is like the water in the Yangtze river, flows to the east fluently. Originated from Yongquan cavity, and (its) path passes the spine on the back. Arrives to the Niwan Gong (i.e., brain), and returns to the Yintang palace. (Use) the Xin (i.e., emotional mind) and Yi (i.e., wisdom mind) to lead the Qi, never apart slightly. For example, when the right fist raises (i.e., emits), the Yi and Qi arrive to the shoulder and armpit. Yi and Qi arrive, the Jin follows, and feels at the inner elbow. Following the opportunity to emit a reverse fist and the Qi reaches the Neiguan cavity. Push to emit the right fist forward, the palm center is slightly jutted out. The Qi reaches the five finger tips along the Yin side of the palm. It is all the same with single or double and there is no difference for hand and feet. (If you) are able to raise one corner, respond with three corners.

氣如長江水，滔滔向東流。來自湧泉穴，
路經脊背過。來到泥丸宮，回到印堂關。
心意將氣領，從不稍離別。譬如右手舉，
意氣到臂腋。隨勁意氣到，覺之在肘窩。
順勢一反拳，氣到內關穴。右拳前按出，
掌心微突越。氣經陰掌面，直到五指尖。
單雙皆一樣，手足無二般。只能舉一隅，
應以三隅反。

The circulation of Qi should be smooth and abundant, like the water flowing in the Yangtze river (i.e., Chang Jiang, 長江). The Yongquan (K-1)(湧泉) cavity is located in the center of the foot, two thirds up from your heel. Since Taiji Jin originates from the feet (i.e., root), the Qi starts from here. Niwan Gong means "mud pill palace," and is a Daoist term that implies the brain or Upper Dan Tian. The author of this poem believes that the Qi streams inward from the bottom of the feet and circulates upward through the spine and then reaches to the Upper Dan Tian (Shang Dan Tian, 上丹田) and finally to the Yintang (M-HN-3)(印堂) palace (i.e., third eye). It is believed that the residence of the Spirit is at the Upper Dan Tian (i.e., brain) and exits and enters from the crown of the head and the third eye.

Xin is an emotional mind, which is Yang and makes you excited, and Yi is a wisdom mind, which is Yin and makes you calm. If you desire to raise up the Spirit of Vitality, you must use the Yang force of Xin to raise, and use the Yin force of Yi to control. In Daoist society, Xin is compared to a monkey while Yin is compared to a horse. The monkey is excited and unstable, while the horse is calm, controlled, and powerful. It is said: "use the Yi horse to control the monkey Xin." This is a method of regulating the mind in meditation.

When you decide to move, the Xin and Yi are generated and this idea immediately leads the Qi to the physical body for power manifestation. If you decide to use your right arm, immediately the mind leads the Qi to the arms. The Neiguan (P-6)(內關) cavity is a major cavity located at the inner side of the forearm near the wrist area. This cavity belongs to the Pericardium Qi channel, which is used to regulate the heart fire. When you decide to lead the Qi to the hands for a strike, the Qi immediately reaches this cavity to energize the arms.

When you use the palm to strike, settle your wrist (i.e., center of palm is jutted out) to manifest the power strongly. The Qi reaches the hands and legs from three Yin primary Qi channels to both your hands and legs. Once you know how the Qi flows in just one of the four limbs, you have already discovered the other three.

Follow this and train continuously, the entire body is threaded as one. Xin and Yi to lead the Qi and Li (i.e., Jin), the limbs and the body move perfectly. Once move, nothing is not moving and once calm, all calm. Once fast, nothing is not fast, once slow, all slow.

Exhalation (the lungs) closes to emit and exit (the Jin) and inhalation (the lungs) opens (and the Qi) returns to the (Lower) Dan Tian. Transport (the Qi) as passing the nine-curved pearl, everywhere is transported (i.e., reached) completely. Do remember do not transport too fast and jump from (Lower) Dan Tian through the spine and reach the finger tips. Without passing every point step by step (i.e., gradually) and without passing individual gates (i.e., cavity). Must walk (i.e., transport) following the steps, the internal and external are naturally harmonized. Xin, Yi, and Li are regulated harmoniously, after long practice, (the Qi) will naturally pass through all gates (i.e., cavities). One year after one year, (you will) become a metal and iron Luo Han (i.e., arhan).

照此練下去，周身一線穿。心意導氣力，
肢體動周全。一動無不動，一靜俱寂然。
一快無不快，一慢皆遲緩。呼合發放出，
吸開歸丹田。行如九曲珠，處處運周全。
切忌行太速，田脊跳指尖。未經步步點，
未經各各關。定要按步走，內外合天然。
心意力調合，久練自過關。一年復一年，
金鋼鐵羅漢。

Follow the key of using the mind to lead the Qi to the arms for Jin manifestation. Remember that the entire body should be connected like ancient Chinese coins threaded together. According to the Chinese definition, Jin means Qi-Li (氣力) or Li-Qi (力氣). This means to use the Qi to energize the muscle to increase the manifested power. Once you are in a situation, remain calm so you can use your calm and strong mind to lead the Qi. If you remain still, the entire body is still and if you decide to act, the entire body acts as one unit. It is the same for developing speed, decided by the mind and corresponding naturally and immediately with the body.

When you exhale (i.e., lungs are closed), the Jin is emitted and when you inhale (i.e., lungs are opened), lead the Qi back to the Lower Dan Tian. Transport the Qi to even the tiniest places of the body.

However, when learning how to use the mind to lead the Qi, you should practice gradually. In order to lead the Qi efficiently and abundantly, you must learn "Small Circulation" and "Grand Circulation" meditation. In these trainings, you must learn to keep the mind, Qi, and breathing harmonized so that the Jin can be manifested powerfully. Once you have reached this stage, you will become a Luo Han (羅漢). Luo Han means arhan, and is the perfect man of Hinayana in Buddhism.

Additional Notes:

Yi (mind) and Qi are the master (sovereign), and the bones and muscles are the chancellor. The waist and the legs are the commanding generals, the palms are the vanguards, and the eyes and skin are the detectors. The master commands and the chancellor follows (the order), the general commands and the vanguards follow. The detectors report to the general with speed and the general reports to the chancellor. The master and the subordinates mutually rely on (each other) and the top and the bottom mutually follow. The entire body (acts) with one Qi.

意氣為君，骨肉為臣。腰腿為主帥，手掌為先鋒，
眼神皮膚為偵探。君令臣使，將令君使。偵探速報
與軍將，軍將命令與臣君。主從相依，上下相隨，
渾身一氣。

Yi (wisdom mind) and Qi always work together. When the mind is generated, the Qi immediately circulates to energize the physical body (i.e., bones and muscles). Therefore, Yi and Qi are like the sovereign in a country and the bones and muscles are the chancellor. Once the action is commanded, the Jin is generated from the legs and con-

trolled by the waist, which governs the power and the ways of manifestation. Therefore, legs and waist are the generals. When this Jin is
manifested to the palms, the palms reach the opponent. The palms
are soldiers, encountering the opponent is the battlefield. However,
the eyes (i.e., first contact by looking) and the skin (i.e., first contact
by feeling) are the intelligence gatherers that collect information on
the opponent and report to the general. All parts rely on one another
for survival, and submit to one another when necessary. Therefore,
the entire body acts as one unit from internal to external and from the
top to the bottom.

Song of Random Circle[13]

Li, Yi-Yu

乱環歌 李亦畬

In (the applications of) round, (it) is as big as heaven and earth, the adhering is as long as the sun and moon. (There are) hundreds of variations in Yin and Yang, the disappearing and the growth of the hardness and softness are following naturally. (Even) adhering is also circling, within the random circling, (there is) no losing (contact) and resistance. Advance the legs following the hands' (techniques), the waist and the legs are the total control.

圓裡乾坤大，沾沾日月長。陰陽百變化，
剛柔任消長。沾沾亦是圈，亂環無丢抗。
腳隨手進步，腰腿全主張。

The theory and applications of round (i.e., Taiji Yin and Yang symbol) can be as abundant and large as the universe (i.e., heaven and earth). Once you know how to stick and adhere with the opponent, you can stay in contact with your opponent for a long time, implying even days or months (i.e., sun and moon). From this Taiji Yin and Yang theory, countless applications can be derived. Additionally, the soft (i.e., Yin) and hard (i.e., Yang) follow each other smoothly and naturally. Once you have mastered the key secret of the round and the Yin and Yang exchange, your adhering will become skillful, and stay in the circle of rounding Yin and Yang. When this happens, you will not lose contact with your opponent, and will not have any resistance or coarseness in moving. The leg stepping follows the techniques and strategies, instead of the techniques and the strategies following the leg movements.

Up and bottom mutually follow and coordinate (harmonious), the applications and the variations are on the two palms. Front and rear as well as left and right, must be carefully and clearly following the opportunity. (When) emitting the palms to touch the (opponent's) chest, (it will be hard) to resist with (the applications of) random circle. Move and shake the opponent's foundation (i.e., root), to emit the sole Qi and reach far distance.

上下相隨和，運化在兩掌。前後與左右，
隨機任端詳。出掌摸前胸，亂環勢難擋。
動搖敵根本，一發氣遠揚。

In order to be round, the top (i.e., Yang) and the bottom (i.e., Yin) must be coordinated harmoniously. Only then can the applications of the palms be various, and the Jin manifested be smooth and powerful. Left (i.e., Yin) and right (i.e., Yang), rear (i.e., Yin) and front (i.e., Yang) must also cooperate with each other. Once you have grasped the application secret of this Yin and Yang Taiji circle, the techniques emitted to the opponent through the hands will be hard to escape. With the power manifested from these Yin and Yang applications, you can pull the opponent's root and bounce him a far distance.

If the opponent uses the upraising hands, Cai (i.e., pluck) and An (i.e., push) are not leaving the path. If the opponent uses An (i.e., push) to press down, follow the downward motion and then raise it up. (If) I am on the top, do not forget to pluck (Cai), (if I am) on the opponent's side, (I) will be busy in sealing and closing. Left and right do not have mistake, emit (my) hands to demonstrate the strength of (my) high skill. Taiji is really a marvelousness, (it) is the king of the random circle.

敵若用挑手，採按不離行。敵若手按下，
隨下再升堂。我上莫忘採，敵旁封閉忙，
左右無參差，出手顯高強。太極真立妙，
亂環術中王。

Cai and An are the two effective techniques to deal with the opponent's upraising hands. When the opponent is raising your arm upward to expose a vital area for an attack, you must use Cai to pluck it down, and follow with An to push him off balance. This will stop him from attempting to raise your arm upward. However, if the opponent uses An to press your arm downward to expose your head and neck for a strike, you should not resist and try to raise it up. Instead, you should first follow his downward motion to yield and neutralize the incoming force, and then immediately follow with an upward raising action to expose his vital areas for your attack.

Whenever your hands are on top of your opponent's hands, you should immediately use Cai to pluck his wrist or elbow downward, so you can expose his head and neck for your attack. However, if you are situated on his side, you should immediately seal and lock his arms to immobilize his further action. Left hand and right hand handle either side of the opponent, all the same. They skillfully cooperate with each other naturally and harmoniously. All success in applying the techniques depends on the marvelous theory and applications of the random circle (i.e., Taiji Yin and Yang symbol).

The Acclamation of Taiji Sparring[13]

Li, Yi-Yu

太極散手贊 李亦畬

The ancestor teacher passed down to us the real marvelous techniques. Hard-soft and insubstantial-substantial are exchangeable according to the opportunity. Within these (techniques), there are a few sayings (we must) ponder profoundly (i.e., carefully). External and internal, coarse and refined always ask the original root (i.e., the cause and the reason). When the opponent wishes to come (i.e., attack), I lead (the coming force) into (the emptiness). When the opponent wishes to exit (i.e., retreat), I drive (him) out as a cow. (If) within the insubstantial, there is no substantial, then (this insubstantial) is not an insubstantial. (If) within the substantial, there is no insubstantial, then (this substantial) is in vain.

祖師傳我真妙法，剛柔虛實隨機變。
個中有語細參求，表裡精粗問根由。
彼欲來時我引進，彼欲出時我逐牛。
虛中無實不為虛，實中無虛枉出頭。

Soft and hard, insubstantial and substantial are classified as Yin and Yang in Taijiquan. They are exchangeable smoothly following the situation. Within the Yin there is Yang and within the Yang there is Yin. Yin is originated from Yang, and Yang is derived from Yin. When the opponent is Yang (i.e., attacks), you react with Yin, and when the opponent is Yin (i.e., retreats), you respond with Yang (i.e., attack). Once you have grasped the trick and skill of Yin and Yang exchange, you can master the essence of Taijiquan.

In the insubstantial, (the techniques) vary following the opportunity (i.e., situation). The marvelous (tricks) are found in the round. When (opponent applies) Ji (i.e., press), Lu (i.e., rollback) can be used to neutralize. When (it is) urgently closed, use Lie (i.e., split) hands (i.e., technique)(to save the urgency). Cai (i.e., pluck) and An (i.e., push) are mutually varied from each other. Offense and defense have their reasons. Entire body (acts) as sole Qi. (It is) abundant as a Taiji ball. There is leading and entering everywhere and there are hands around the entire body. (If) offense and defense are not discriminated clearly, (the applications of) the insubstantial and substantial are not reliable. It is like a moon in Zhong Yuan festival (i.e., mid-August of Chinese calendar), its shining reaches the nine continents (i.e., everywhere). Once (you) have trained and reached to the insubstantial and empty place (i.e., so natural and hard to see your intention), (you) will be (in the state) of no offense and defense.

虛中隨機變，妙在圓中求。擠時可攦化，
迫近出挒手。採按互變化，功守有來由。
周身如一氣，渾如太極球。處處有引進，
滿身都是手。攻守不分明，虛實無憑證。
恍如中元月，光霞照九州。練到虛無處，
無攻亦無守。

When you are in the insubstantial situation, you may remain insubstantial or change into substantial depending on the situation. The exchange should be smooth and natural as a Taiji ball (i.e., round). If the opponent uses Ji against me (i.e., substantial), immediately use Lu (i.e., insubstantial) to neutralize the incoming Ji. If the opponent is urgently close (i.e., substantial), step to the side to avoid the incoming attack (i.e., insubstantial), and immediately use Lie to bounce him off balance (i.e., substantial). Cai is insubstantial while An is substantial. Both are used together. Normally, right after Cai, apply An immediately.

Leading is insubstantial while entering is substantial. Skillfully exchange insubstantial and substantial with both hands. It seems these two hands are everywhere around both your body and your opponent's. However, insubstantial and substantial should be clearly executed. To do something halfway is not complete, and therefore not effective. In addition, it will give your opponent a chance to escape and catch the opportunity to attack you. The techniques are performed clearly as the Zhong Yuan (中元) moon, shining and bright. The Zhong Yuan festival is the Chinese Ghost Festival on the 15th night of the seventh moon. On this night, the moon is round and shines very brightly.

If you can comprehend the theory and master the applications of Yin and Yang, once you have reached to a very high level, you will reach the stage called "the fight of no fight." This means that all of your reactions become supremely natural and smooth. Your mind reacts naturally and with complete neutrality.

References

1. "太極拳，刀、劍、桿、散手合編" (*Tai Chi Chuan: Saber, Sword, Staff, and Sparring*), Chen, Yan-Lin (陳炎林), Reprinted in Taipei, Taiwan, 1943.

2. 太極拳講義，吳公藻編，上海書店，1985.

3. 南雷集王征南墓誌銘：〝宋之張三豐為武當丹士。徽宗召之，路梗不得進。夜夢元帝授之拳法，厥明以單丁殺賊百餘。〞

4. 明史方妓傳：〝張三豐遼東懿州人，名全一。一名君寶。三豐其號也。以不修邊幅，又號張邋遢。頎而偉，龜形鶴背。大耳圓目，鬚髯如戟。寒暑惟一衲蓑，所啖升斗輒盡。或數日不食，或數月不食，一日千里。善嬉戲，旁若無人。嘗與其徒遊武當。築草廬而居之，洪武二十四年，太祖聞其名，遣使覓之不得。〞

5. 明郎瑛七修類稿：〝張仙名君寶，字全一。別號玄玄，時人又稱張邋遢。天順三年，曾來謁帝。予見其像，鬚鬢豎立，一髻背垂，紫面大腹，而攜笠者。上為錫誥之文，封為通微顯化真人。〞

6. 太極拳全書，人民體育出版社，1988.

7. 太極拳術，顧留馨著，上海體育出版社，1992.

8. 楊禹廷太極系列秘要集錦，李秉慈、翁福麒編著，奧林匹克出版社，1990.

9. 逸民氏《陰符槍譜·序》：〝山右王先生，自少時經史而外，黃帝、老子之書及兵家言，無書不讀，而兼通擊刺之術，槍法其尤精者也。〞

10. *The History of Chinese Wushu*, Lin, Bo-Yuan, 1996, Wu Zhou Publications, Taipei. (中國武術史，五洲出版社，臺北。)

11. *Tai Chi Theory & Martial Power*, Dr. Yang, Jwing-Ming, YMAA, 1996.

12. *Lost Tai-Chi Classics from the Late Ch'ing Dynasty*, Douglas Wile, 1996.

13. *Chinese Wushu Great Dictionary*, 1990, (中國武術大辭典，人民體育出版社。).

Appendix: Translation and Glossary of Chinese Terms

An 按

One of the Taijiquan basic thirteen postures. An means "to push" or "press down." Often, it is also used as push forward or upward.

Ba Men 八門

Means "eight doors." Taijiquan is constructed out of thirteen basic postures, which include eight basic body movement patterns and five stepping strategies. The right basic body movements are commonly compared to the eight trigrams in Baguazhgang, and are called the "eight doors."

Bai He 白鶴

Means "White Crane." One of the Chinese southern martial styles.

Cai 採

"Plucking."

Chan 纏

"To wrap" or "to coil." A common Chinese martial arts technique.

Chan Si Jin 纏絲勁

"Silk Reeling Jin." An inner coiling Jin training in Taijiquan.

Chang Chuan (Changquan) 長拳

Means "Long Range Fist." Chang Chuan includes all northern Chinese long range martial styles.

Chang Jiang 長江

Literally, "long river." Refers to the Yangtze river in southern China.

Changquan (Chang Chuan) 長拳

Means "Long Range Fist." Changquan includes all northern Chinese long range martial styles.

Cheng, Gin-Gsao (1911-1976)

Dr. Yang, Jwing-Ming's White Crane master.

Chi (Qi) 氣

The energy pervading the universe, including the energy circulating in the human body.

Chi Kung (Qigong) 氣功

The Gongfu of Qi, which means the study of Qi.

Chin Na (Qin Na) 擒拿

Literally means "grab control." A component of Chinese martial arts which emphasizes grabbing techniques, to control your opponent's joints, in conjunction with attacking certain acupuncture cavities.

Confucius 孔子

A Chinese scholar, during the period of 551-479 B.C., whose philosophy has significantly influenced Chinese culture.

Da 打

"To strike." Normally, to attack with the palms, fists or arms.

Da Zhou Tian 大周天

Literally, "Grand Cycle Heaven." Usually translated Grand Circulation. After a Nei Dan Qigong practitioner completes Small Circulation, he will circulate his Qi through the entire body or exchange the Qi with nature.

Dan Tian 丹田

"Elixir Field." Located in the lower abdomen. It is considered the place which can store Qi energy.

Dang 檔

Inner thigh area.

Dao 道

The "way," by implication the "natural way."

Dazhui (Gv-14) 大椎

One of the acupuncture cavities belonging to the Governing Vessel.

Dian Xue 點穴

Dian means "to point and exert pressure" and Xue means "the cavities." Dian Xue refers to those Qin Na techniques which specialize in attacking acupuncture cavities to immobilize or kill an opponent.

Dian Xue Massages 點穴按摩

One of Chinese massage techniques in which the acupuncture cavities are stimulated through pressing. Dian Xue massage is also called acupressure and is the root of Japanese Shiatsu.

Dong Jin 懂勁

"Understanding Jin." It means to understand one's own Jin and also the opponent's Jin.

Du Mai 督脈

Usually translated "Governing Vessel." One of the eight extraordinary vessels.

Gong Qiao 拱橋

Means "arcing bridge" in Chinese martial arts society.

Gongfu (Kung Fu) 功夫

Means "energy-time." Anything which will take time and energy to learn or to accomplish is called Gongfu.

Gu 顧

"Beware of." It means to beware of the left in Taijiquan.

Guoshu 國術

Abbreviation of "Zhongguo Wushu," which means "Chinese Martial Techniques."

Haidi 海底

Means "Sea Bottom." This is a name given by martial artists to the Huiyin cavity (Co-1) in Chinese medicine. Perineum.

Han, Ching-Tang 韓慶堂

A well known Chinese martial artist, especially in Taiwan in the last forty years. Master Han is also Dr. Yang, Jwing-Ming's Long Fist Grand Master.

Henan 河南省

The province in China where the Shaolin Temple is located.

Huang Ting 黃庭

Literally, "yellow yard." It implies the area called "Jade Ring" in Daoist society. The area is located at the solar plexus.

Huiyin (Co-1) 會陰

One of the acupuncture cavities belonging to the Conception Vessel.

Ji 擠

Means "to squeeze" or "to press."

Jin Bu 進步

"Step forward." Taijiquan is constructed from thirteen basic postures, which include basic moving patterns and strategic steppings. Jin Bu is one of the five steppings.

Jin (Jing) 勁

Chinese martial power. A combination of "Li" (muscular power) and "Qi."

Jin, Shao-Feng 金紹峰

Dr. Yang, Jwing-Ming's White Crane grand master.

Jing (Jin) 勁

Chinese martial power. A combination of "Li" (muscular power) and "Qi."

Jing-Shen 精神

Literally, "essential spirit." The meaning is the spirit of vitality.

Kao 靠

Means "bump." One of the Taijiquan thirteen postures.

Kao, Tao 高濤

Master Yang, Jwing-Ming's first Taijiquan master.

Kong Men 空門

"Empty door." Means an empty space which allows the opponent to enter.

Kua 胯

Inner thigh area.

Kung (Gong) 功

Means "energy" or "hard work."

Kung Fu (Gongfu) 功夫

Means "energy-time." Anything which will take time and energy to learn or to accomplish is called Kung Fu.

Li 力

The power which is generated from muscular strength.

Li, Mao-Ching 李茂清

Dr. Yang, Jwing-Ming's Long Fist master.

Li, Yi-Yu (1832-1892 A.D.) 李亦畬

Also named Li, Jing-Lun. He was Wŭ, Cheng-Qing's student, and also his nephew. He also learned from Wŭ, Yu-Xiang.

Li-Qi 力氣

When you use Li (muscular power) you also need Qi to support it. However, when this Qi is led by a concentrated mind, the Qi is able to manifest the muscular power to a higher level and is therefore called Jin. Li-Qi (or Qi-Li) is a general definition of Jin and commonly implies manifested power.

Lie 挒

"Split" or "rend." One of the thirteen basic postures in Taijiquan.

Lu 擺

"Rollback." One of the thirteen basic postures in Taijiquan.

Luo Han 羅漢

Luo Han means arhan, and is the perfect man of Hinayana in Buddhism.

Mingmen (Gv-4) 命門

One of the acupuncture cavities belonging to the Governing Vessel.

Na 拿

Means "to hold" or "to grab." Also an abbreviation for Chin Na, or Qin Na.

Nei Gong 內功

Internal Gongfu. This implies those practices which involve internal Qi training.

Nei Jin 內勁

Internal Jin, which means the capability of using the mind to lead the Qi.

Nei Jin Li 內勁力

When the mind leads the Qi to the physical body and manifests it to power it is called Nei Jin Li.

Neiguan (P-6) 內關

One of the acupuncture cavities belonging to the Pericardium Primary Qi Channel.

Pan 盼

"Look." It means to look to the right in Taijiquan.

Peng 掤

"Wardoff." One of the Taijiquan basic thirteen postures.

Qi (Chi) 氣

Chinese term for universal energy. A current popular model is that the Qi circulating in the human body is bioelectric in nature.

Qi-Li 氣力

Qi that has been manifested into Li. This means Jin.

Qigong (Chi Kung) 氣功

The Gongfu of Qi, which means the study of Qi.

Qin (Chin) 擒

Means "to catch" or "to seize."

Qin Na (Chin Na) 擒拿

Literally means "grab control." A component of Chinese martial arts which emphasizes grabbing techniques to control your opponent's joints, in conjunction with attacking certain acupuncture cavities.

Shang Dan Tian 上丹田

Upper Dan Tian. Located at the third eye, it is the residence of the Shen (spirit).

Shaolin 少林

"Young woods." Name of the Shaolin Temple.

Shaolin Temple 少林寺

A monastery located in Henan Province, China. The Shaolin Temple is well known because of its martial arts training.

Shen 神

"Spirit." According to Chinese Qigong, the Shen resides at the Upper Dan Tian (the third eye).

Shuai 摔

Means "to throw." An abbreviation of "Shuai Jiao" (wrestling).

Shuai Jiao 摔跤

Chinese wrestling. Part of Chinese martial arts.

Tai Chi Chuan (Taijiquan) 太極拳

A Chinese internal martial style which is based on the theory of Taiji (grand ultimate).

Taiji 太極

Means "Grand Ultimate." It is this force which generates two poles, Yin and Yang.

Taiji Qigong 太極氣功

A Qigong training specially designed for Taijiquan practice.

Taijiquan (Tai Chi Chuan) 太極拳

A Chinese internal martial style which is based on the theory of Taiji (grand ultimate).

Taipei 台北

The capital city of Taiwan located in the north.

Taiwan 台灣

An island to the south-east of mainland China. Also known as "Formosa."

Taiwan University 台灣大學

A well-known university located in northern Taiwan.

Taizuquan 太祖拳

A southern style of Chinese external martial arts.

Tamkang 淡江

Name of a University in Taiwan.

Tamkang College Guoshu Club 淡江國術社

A Chinese martial arts club
founded by Dr. Yang when he was studying in Tamkang University.

Ti 踢

Means "to kick."

Ting Jin 聽勁

"Listening Jin." It means the sensitivity of feeling or sensing in Taijiquan.

Tu 土

"Earth." One of the five elements.

Tui 退

"Retreat."

Tui Bu 退步

"Step Backward." One of the Taijiquan thirteen postures. Taijiquan is constructed from eight basic moving patterns (eight doors) and five strategic steppings (five steppings). Tui Bu is one of the five steppings.

Tui Na 推拿

Means "to push and grab." A category of Chinese massages for healing and injury treatment.

Wai Jin 外勁

External power. The type of Jin where the muscles predominate and only local Qi is used to support the muscles.

Wang, Zong-Yue 王宗岳

A well-known Chinese Taijiquan master during the Qing Qian Long Period (1736–1796 A.D.).

Wei Qi 衛氣

Protective Qi or Guardian Qi. The Qi at the surface of the body which generates a shield to protect the body from negative external influences such as colds.

Weilu 尾閭

Tailbone.

Wilson Chen 陳威伸

Dr. Yang, Jwing-Ming's friend.

Wu Gong 五弓

Five bows. Taijiquan considers there to be five bows in the human body, which allows you to store and then emit power. The two arms and two legs are four bows, while the torso is one bow.

Wu Style Taijiquan 吳氏太極拳

A Taijiquan style created by Wu, Quan-You (1834-1902 A.D.).

Wŭ Style Taijiquan 武氏太極拳

A Taijiquan style created by Wŭ, Yu-Xiang (1812-1880 A.D.).

Wŭ, Cheng-Qing 武澄清

A well-known Taijiquan master during the 19th century. Wŭ, Yu-Xiang's oldest brother.

Wŭ, Yu-Xiang (1812-1880 A.D.) 武禹襄

Also named He-Qing. He learned Taijiquan Chen style old posture from Yang, Lu-Shan, and also Chen style new posture from Chen, Qing-Ping.

Wuji 無極

Means "no extremity."

Wushu 武術

Literally, "martial techniques."

Xia Dan Tian 下丹田

Lower Dan Tian. Located in the lower abdomen, it is believed to be the residence of water Qi (Original Qi).

Xiao Zhou Tian 小周天

Literally, small heavenly cycle. Also called Small Circulation. In Qigong, when you can use your mind to lead Qi through the Conception and Governing Vessels, you have completed "Xiao Zhou Tian."

Xin 心

Means "heart." Xin means the mind generated from emotional disturbance.

Xinzhu Xian 新竹縣

Birthplace of Dr. Yang, Jwing-Ming in Taiwan.

Yan Lo 閻羅王

The king who is in charge of Hell.

Yang 陽

Too sufficient. One of the two poles. The other is Yin.

Yang, Lu-Chan (1799-1872) 楊露禪

Also named Fu-Kuai. The
creator of Yang style Taijiquan.

Yang, Jwing-Ming 楊俊敏

Author of this book.

Yi 意

Wisdom mind. The mind generated from wise judgment.

Yi Jing 易經

Book of Changes. A book of divination written during the Zhou
Dynasty (1122-255 B.C.).

Yi Shou Dan Tian 意守丹田

Keep your Yi on your Lower Dan Tian. In Qigong training, you
keep your mind at the Lower Dan Tian in order to build up Qi.
When you are circulating your Qi, you always lead your Qi back
to your Lower Dan Tian before you stop.

Yin 陰

Deficient. One of the two poles. The other is Yang.

Yintang (M-HN-3) 印堂

An acupuncture cavity belonging to miscellaneous cavities.

Yongquan (K-1) 湧泉

Bubbling Well. Name of an acupuncture cavity belonging to the
Kidney Primary Qi Channel.

You Pan 右盼

"Look to the Right." One of the Taijiquan thirteen postures.

Yu Huan Xue 玉環穴

Jade ring cavity. It means the space inside the solar plexus area.

Zhan Jin 粘勁

Adhering Jin.

Zhang Jin 長勁

Growing Jin.

Zhang, Xiang-San 張祥三

A well known Chinese martial artist in Taiwan.

Zhong Ding 中定

"Firm the Center." One of the Taijiquan thirteen postures.

Zhong Gong 中宮

Central palace. The space between the legs.

Zhong Guo Wushu 中國武術

Chinese Wushu.

Zhong Ting 中庭

Central yard, also called jade ring. The inner space behind the solar plexus.

Zhou 肘

"Elbow." To use the elbow to execute defensive or offensive techniques in Taijiquan.

Index

Abdominal Breathing (Reverse), 40
Adhere, 15, 31-35, 47, 49, 61, 66, 73, 82, 84, 97
Advance (Jin), 25, 28, 35, 42
   see also Advance and retreat
Advance and retreat, 43, 44
Aggressive, 85
Agile, 21, 26, 33, 49, 54, 55, 70
Agitated, see Qi, 72
Alert, 82
Alignment, 85
Alive, 2, 21, 26, 45, 54, 75, 83
An (Push), 31, 35, 76, 79, 84, 98, 102
Angling, 77, 79
Anus, see Huiyin cavity
Arcing Bridge, see Bridging Hands
Arcing, see Torso, Back, Chest, Arms
Arms, 64, 85
Attach, 54
Attack,
   the appearance of the attack, 4
   timing, see Timing
Attention, see Yi, see also Broken Jin, under Jin
Awareness, see Spirit of Vitality
Back, 21, 25, 43, 44, 69, 70, 80
Balance, 26, 45, 63, 64, 70, 80, 83, 84, 86
   balancing the upward Qi, 40
   unbalancing the opponent, see Opponent
   Yin and Yang balancing, 64
Bending (Storing), 35, 39, 41, 43, 44, 56, 57
Bending the elbow(s), see Elbow
Beware of the Left (Gu), 35, 78, 80
Body, 9, 10, 64
Bone Marrow Breathing, 63
Bone Marrow, see Condensing Qi and Spirit
Bones, 94, 95
Book of Changes, see *Yi Jing*
Borrow opponent's energy, 59
Borrow opponent's Li, 49, 56, 58
Bottom of the feet, see Yongquan
Bows for storing and emitting Jin, 17, 19, 26, 50
Breathing, 7, 11, 12, 55, 56
Bridging Hands, 83
Bump, see Kao
Cai (Pluck), 35, 76, 77, 81, 82, 84, 86, 88, 89, 98, 99, 102
Calmness, 4, 9, 10, 50, 53, 54, 64, 66, 72, 93
Cartwheel(s), 25, 29, 40, 45, 54
Cavities,
   exposing the opponent's cavities, 76, 77, 99
   Qi passing through all the cavities, 93
   striking cavities, 2, 3, 17, 18, 51
Center, 21, 26, 63, 64, 70, 80, 85, 89
Center Door, 78, 86, 87
Central Equilibrium (Zhong Ding or Tu), 35, 36, 78, 82, 85, 86

Central Palace, see Zhong Gong
Chancellor, 94, 95
Chest
   bow for storing/emitting Jin, 17, 64, 71
   swallow, draw in, contain the chest, 21, 25, 26, 43, 44, 69, 70, 78, 80
Chin Na, see Qin Na
Circles, 8, 97
Close range, 79, 102
Closing, 58, 59, 64, 66, 67, 93
Clumsiness, 2, 24, 40, 51, 54, 71, 87
Coiling, 57, 69
Comfort, 26
Commanding generals, 94
Concentration, 6, 53, 63
Condensing the Qi, 49, 50, 63
Condensing the Spirit, see Spirit
Connect, 35, 36
Connected, see Unit
Connection areas, 65, 70
Continuity of the Yi, 6
Continuity, 4
Controlling the opponent, 54, 55
Coordinating,
   legs, waist, arms, 82, 85
   upper and lower body/internal and external, 36, 37, 94, 95, 98
Counterattack (avoiding), 89
Cover, 14, 19
Crotch, 21, 88, 89
Crown of the head (Baihui), 92
Curved, see Bending
Da (striking), 17, 18, 84, 85
Dan Tian,
   generating Qi at the Lower Dan Tian, 5, 26
   leading Qi from Lower Dan Tian, 72
   sinking/storing Qi in Lower Dan Tian, v, viii, 2, 5, 21, 25, 26, 39, 40, 42, 44, 50, 56-59, 63, 69, 70, 93, 94
   Upper Dan Tian, see Brain
Dao, 23, 40, 41, 69
Daoist Qigong, 69
Dazhui (Gv-14), 19
Defense, 83, 102
Deflecting the attack, 49
Door, see Empty Door and Center Door
Double Weighting (resisting), 29, 41, 42, 44, 63, 66, 67, 72
Draw in, 58, 59
Drum (Dan Tian taut like a drum), 59, 62
Du mai, see Governing Vessel
Earth (Five Elements), 80
Eight Directions, 2, 3, 25, 45
Elbow(s)
   Bending the elbow(s), 43

Elbow Jin, see Zhou
Elbows not past the knee, 84, 85
Sink/Drop the elbows, 21, 63, 69, 70, 76, 77
Emitting Jin, see Jin
Emotional Mind, see Xin
Empty Door, 79
Enlightenment, 14, 46, 47
Entering, 102
Entwining, see Mutual Entwining
Exchanging Hands, see Sparring
Exchanging Soft and Hard, see Soft and Hard
Exhale, 93
Exposing the opponent, 49, 99
    see also Opponent
Extending (Emitting), 35, 41, 43
Extending the tendons, see Tendons
External and Internal harmonized, 93-95
External dynamic force, see Li
External expression of the Internal, 10, 11, 32, 63, 70, 71
External Jin, see Wai Jin
External muscular strength: see Li
Eyes, 94, 95
Fast, 49, 72
Feeling, see Listening Jin
Feet (Root), 56, 57, 64, 70, 71
Fight of No Fight, 41, 102, 103
Fighting Spirit, 71
Fighting strategy in Taiji, 6
Fighting, 65
Fingers (expressing Jin), 56, 70, 71, 93
Five Elements, 80
Five Steppings, 35
Fluidity, 4
Folding, 6, 7
Follow the opportunity, 98, 101, 102
Follow, 15, 27, 29, 31, 35, 36, 41-44, 46, 47, 49, 53-56, 61-63, 66, 72, 73, 76, 88, 99
Footwork in Taijiquan, 5, 6
Force against force, see Double Weighting
Four ounces repel one thousand pounds, 9, 24, 32, 36, 37, 56, 61, 62, 64, 65, 72, 73
Front and rear, 98
Full, see Qi
Generals, 94, 95
Give up yourself, 54, 62
Gong Qiao (Arcing Bridge), see Bridging Hands
Governing Vessel, 19
Grand Circulation, 19, 94
Grand Ultimate, 44
Growing Jin, 28
Guardian Qi, see Wei Qi
Half step, 78, 79
Hands, 57, 71, 99
Hanging the crotch, see Crotch
Hardness, 39, 71, 97, 101
Harmonizing mind, Qi and breathing, 94

Harmonizing top and bottom, 98
Head, 2, 25, 43, 44, 69, 70
Heart Fire, regulating, 92
Heart Mind, see Xin
Heart Mind, see Xin
Heaviness, 2
Heng Jin, see Sideways Power
Hips, 21, 25, 43, 44
Hip joints, 65
Hou Tui, see Step Back
Hua Jin, see Neutralizing Jin
Huang Ting, see Jade Ring
Huiyin (cavity)(Co-1), 21
Immobilizing the opponent, see Opponent
Inhalation, 93, 94
Insubstantial,
    see also Yin and Yang
    an insubstantial energy leads the head upward, v, 2, 25
    substantial and insubstantial, v, viii, 2, 25, 28, 35, 36, 40-42, 54-57, 65, 71, 101-103
Intercept, 66
Internal Jin, see Nei Jin
Internal organs
Internal, see External
    shocking the internal organs, 18, 51
Jade Ring, 69
Ji (Press), 35, 75, 76, 77, 81-84, 102
Jin,
    applying Jin, 11
    broken Jin (restoring), 6, 9, 41
    different kinds of Jins, 1, 2
    directing Jin, 31
    emitting/manifesting Jin, 2-5, 17-19, 21, 24, 31-40, 42, 50-59, 63-65, 70-73, 85, 92-95, 98
    generating Jin, 31, 71, 95
    Jin is generated from the legs, 95
    Jin is integrated (one unit), 56
    Jin is originated/generated from Xin and Yi, 70, 92
    Jin is originated from the feet, 92
    Jin is straight, not curved, 50
    soft Jin, 17, 18, 50, 51, 71, 85
    storing/accumulating Jin, 4, 5, 17-19, 21, 25, 26, 43, 49, 50, 56, 57, 65
    supporting Jin by Qi, 1, 2, 3, 4, 5, 6, 59
    What is Jin?, 1, 2, 40, 93
    Yi and Qi arrive, Jin follows, 91
Jing-Shen, see Spirit of Vitality
Joint locks, see Qin Na
Juang Zi, 40
Judgment accurate and clear, 72
Kao (Bump), 21, 35, 78, 79, 84-86, 88, 89
Kicking, see Ti
Knowing the opponent, 62, 63, 65-67
Knowing yourself, 65, 66, 67
Kong Men, see Empty Door

Kua, viii, 21, 25, 26, 43, 44
Lao Zi, 40, 41
Leading (into emptiness), 21-28, 32, 36, 37, 41, 42,
   44-46, 49, 54, 61, 66, 72-77, 80-82, 86, 101-103
Leaning, 69, 80, 89
Left and right, 98
Legs
   generating Jin, 51, 57, 85, 94
   using the legs, 70, 97
   varying the strategy of the movement, 64, 97
Li (muscular power), 1, 3, 17, 18, 49, 53, 58, 70,
Li style, v, vii, viii
Li, Jing-Lun, see Li, Yi-Yu
Li, Yi-Yu, vii, xix, xx
Li-Qi, see Jin
Liang, Qiang-Ya, v, vii, viii, ix
Lie (Split), 35, 102
Lie Jin (Split or Diagonal Wardoff), 75, 76, 86, 87
Lightness, 55, 57, 70
Locking, see Qin Na
Long range, 87, 88, 89
Look to the Right (Pan), 35, 78, 80
Looseness, 26, 63, 69
Losing, see No losing
Lower Dan Tian, see Dan Tian
Lu (Rollback), 31, 35, 76, 77, 82-85, 102
Lungs, 93, 94
Luo Han, 93, 94
Listening Jin, 15, 24, 31, 32, 36, 41-44, 47, 49, 54-57,
   61, 62, 64, 66, 73, 75, 76
Manifesting Jin, see Jin
Master,
   Yi and Qi are the master, 94, 95
Match, 14, 19, 49
Measuring the opponent's strength with Peng, 81
Meditation, 92, 94
Mind,
   see also Xin (Emotional Mind) and Yi
      (Wisdom Mind)
   mind corresponding with body, 93
   mind not broken, 9
   mind: Dao of Taijiquan, 24
   regulating the mind, 64, 66, 92
   steadiness of mind, 50
   the mind leads, 8, 9, 10, 12, 19, 42, 54, 58, 59,
      93-95
Mingmen (Gv-4), 6, 19
Moving Patterns, see Thirteen Postures
Mud Pill Palace, see Brain
Muscles, 94, 95
Muscular force, see Li
Nature, natural, 69, 70, 87, 97, 99, 103
Nei Jin (internal Jin), 3, 4, 18, 19, 26, 71
Neiguan cavity (P-6), 91, 92
Neutralize, 21, 24, 27, 29, 32, 36, 39, 41, 44-46, 50,
   57, 59, 61, 63, 65, 75-77, 79-85, 87, 88, 99, 102
Nine-curved hole/pearl, 3, 40, 93

Niwan Gong (Mud Pill Palace or Upper Dan
   Tian), see Brain
No Extremity, see Wuji
No losing, 53, 97
No resisting, 53, 97, 99
Offense, 102
Opening the opponent, 49
Opening, 58, 64, 66, 67, 93
Opponent,
   attacks, 101
   avoiding his Zhou and Kao, 85, 86
   confusing him, 77
   destroying his intention of attacking, 73
   dodges my bump, 89
   exposing his cavities, 76, 79, 99
   grasping his intention, 76
   immobilizing him, 99
   occupying his center door, 78
   opponent solid and strong, 75, 76
   opponent void, 75, 76
   putting him in the defensive, 73, 89
   retreats, 101
   steps back and/or uses Cai, 84, 85, 87
   tricking him, 76
   tries to expose my cavities, 98, 99
   unbalancing him, 77, 78, 79, 81-83, 85, 89, 98,
Palms,
   function, 94, 95
   Spirit and Yi manifested on the palms, 82
Palm strike, 92
Palms are round, 81
Pan, see Look to the Right
Peaceful, see Calm
Penetrating power, 51
Peng Jin, 26, 35, 44, 65, 70, 75-77, 80, 81, 84, 85
Pericardium Qi Channel, 92
Play Guitar, 88
Pluck, see Cai
Post-Heaven Force, 40
Posture(s), 8, 25, 26, 63
Power,
   see also Jin
   how to develop real power, 7, 11, 12, 40
   the soft power of Taiji, 17, 18
Practicing, 65, 66
Press, see Ji
Pulsating energy, 59
Push, see An
Pushing Hands, xi, 83
Qi,
   see also Dan Tian
   circulating Qi throughout the body, 1, 9, 10, 93,
      94
   condensing Qi into the bones/spine, 1, 9, 10,
      50, 55, 58, 62
   coordinating actions with breathing and Qi, 7,
      45, 50, 82

coordinating mind and Qi, 2
developing your Qi, 7, 8, 59
leading the Qi, viii, 72, 92, 93
Qi passing through all the cavities, 93
Qi starts from the feet, 92
regulating the Qi, 11, 12
storing the Qi, 9, 10, 21, 50, 63
the mind leads the Qi, 12, 58, 70, 93, 94
the Qi follows, 72
using Qi to support Jin, 1-5, 50, 56, 82, 93, 98
Xin and Yi lead the Qi, 92
Yi and Qi are the master, 94, 95
Yi and Qi arrive, Jin follows, 91
Qi-Li, see Jin
Qian Jin, see Step Forward
Qigong, xi
Qin Na, xi, 17, 18, 99
Qing Dynasty, v, vii
Quiet, see Calm
Random Circle, 97, 98, 99
Range, see Long range and Short range
Regulating (body, breathing, mind, Qi, Spirit), 40
Regulating the Heart Fire, see Heart Fire
Regulating Xin, Yi and Li harmoniously, 93
Relaxation,
    body relaxed, 26, 45, 64, 70
    reach hardness/power through relaxation/soft-
    ness, 7, 50
Release, 58, 64
Repel, 24, 76
Resisting, see Double Weighting, and No resisting
Restoring broken Jin, see Broken Jin, under Jin
Retreat (Tui), 25, 28, 35, 42, 84, 85, 87
Reverse Abdominal Breathing, see Abdominal
    Breathing
Rollback, see Lu
Root, 21, 26, 44, 45, 51, 56, 57, 63, 64, 70, 77, 80-87,
    92, 98
Rotating the waist, see Waist
Roundness, 2, 39, 75, 97, 98, 102
Scattered Qi, 56
Seal, 87
Sealing the breath, 79, 88
Sealing the opponent, 81, 82, 98, 99
Sealing vital areas, 70
Sense of enemy, 82
Setup,
    for advancing, 44
    for attack, 42
Shang Dan Tian (Upper Dan Tian), see Brain
Shen, see Spirit
Shocking internal organs, see Internal organs
Short range, 87, 88, 89
Shoulder(s),
    bumping with shoulder, see Kao
    drop/relax/sink the shoulders, 21, 45, 63, 69, 70,
    76, 77

function 64, 65
Shuai (wrestling), 17, 18
Sideways Power (Heng Jin), 86, 87
Silk (soft as silk), 69, 70
Sink the elbows, see Elbows
Sink the Qi, see Qi
Sink the shoulders, see Shoulders
Sinking opponent's attack, 73, 83-86
Sinking, 76, 77, 81
Skin Breathing, 63
Skin feeling, see Listening Jin, 41
Skin, 94, 95
Slender, 41, 70
Slow practice, 65, 66
Small Circulation, 94
Softness,
    being soft, 41, 45, 49, 64, 69, 70, 75, 86, 97, 101
    reaching hardness through softness, 7
    using softness against strength, 39, 44
Soldiers, 95
Solid (force), 76, 86
Sovereign, Yi and Qi are the sovereign, 94, 95
Sparring, 31, 32, 33, 43
Speed, 86, 87
Spine, 5, 6, 91, 92
    bow for storing/emitting Jin/Qi, 17, 18 ,19, 50,
    56, 57, 58, 70, 71, 93
Spiral, 69
Spirit,
    condensing the Spirit, 57, 62, 63, 72
    manifestation of the Spirit, 70, 82
    raising the Spirit, 59, 64, 70, 72, 82
    regulating the Spirit, 64
    residence of the Spirit, 92
    Spirit leads and Qi follows, 72
Spirit of fighting, see Fighting Spirit
Spirit of Vitality (Jing-Shen),
    concentrating on, 11, 12
    raising/strengthening, 2, 4, 10, 25, 26, 40, 43, 44,
    55, 56-59, 62, 63, 70, 92
Stableness, 4
Stagnant, 24, 29, 54
Step Back, 79, 80, 84, 85
Step Forward (Qian Jin), 79, 84, 85
Stepping and stepping strategy, 6, 7, 11, 35, 69, 72,
    78, 79, 97
Sticking, 31, 32, 47, 73, 82, 84, 97
Stiff, 29, 49
Storing the Jin, see Jin
Storing the Qi, see Qi and Dan Tian
Straightness, 39, 50, 56, 57
Strategy, 25, 42, 42, 97
Strength, see Li and Power
Stretch the back, see Back
Strike the Coming Jin, 46
Strike the Nascent Jin, 45, 46
Strike the Oppressive Jin, 27

Strike the Returning Jin, 27, 46
Striking Hands, see Sparring and Fighting
Striking, see Da
Substantial and insubstantial, v, viii, 2, 25, 35, 36,
    40, 41, 42, 44, 54, 55, 56, 57, 65, 71, 101, 102,
    see also Yin and Yang
Suffuse (Spread), 13, 19
Sun style Taijiquan, v, vii
Swallow, 14, 15, 19
Swelling, 71
Taiji, 23, 44
Taiji Ball, 102
Tailbone upright, 69, 70
Tendons, 70, 71
Tense, 71, 86
Third Eye, 91, 92
Thirteen Postures/Basic Patterns of Taijiquan, 35,
    37, 41, 75-80
Ti (kicking), 17, 18
Timing your attack/defense, 9, 27, 45, 46, 47, 51,
    56, 57
    see also Strike
Ting Jin, see Listening Jin
Top and bottom, 98
Torso, 17, 18, 19, 21, 71
Tu, see Central Equilibrium
Unbalancing, see Uprooting, Balance and
    Opponent
Understanding Jin, 24, 28, 32, 33, 49, 63
Unification, see Unite
Unit,
    moving as a unit, 10, 37, 45, 51, 54, 57, 62-64,
    69, 70, 72, 85, 92-94, 102
    see also Connection areas
Unite/Unify, 24, 25, 32, 62, 71
Up and Bottom, 98
Upper Dan Tian, see Brain
Upraising hands (exposing vital area), 98, 99
Uprooting, 21
Uprooting/Unbalancing the opponent, 49, 66, 67,
    89, 98
Urgent, 28, 102
Vanguards, 94
Vibrating energy, 59
Void, see Opponent
Wai Jin, 18, 19, 71
Waist,
    rotating the waist, 6, 7, 76
    soften, loosen the waist, 78, 80, 83
    waist directs the Qi, 12
    waist directs/controls the Jin, 31, 32, 44, 51, 56,
    57, 64, 65, 71, 77, 85, 94, 95, 97
    waist leads body, 8, 36, 37, 45, 70, 87, 97
Wang, Zong-Yue, xix, 23, 39
Wardoff Diagonally, see Lie Jin
Wardoff Jin, see Peng Jin
Wei Qi, 13

Weight distribution, 78, 80, 89
Whipping power, see soft Jin, under Jin
Wisdom Mind, see Yi
Withdraw, 59, 64, 65, 89
Wrapping the inner thighs, see Kua
Wrestling, see Shuai
Wrist, 71, 91, 92
Wu Gong (Five Bows), see Bows
Wu style Taijiquan, v, vii
Wŭ style Taijiquan, v, vii, viii
Wŭ, Cheng-Qing, v, vii, xix
Wŭ, He-Qing, see Wŭ, Yu-Xiang
Wŭ, Ru-Qing, v, vii, xix, xx
Wŭ, Yu-Xiang, v, vii, xix, xx
Wu, Quan-You, xix
Wudang Taijiquan, viii
Wuji, 23
Xin (Heart Mind or Emotional Mind),
    see also Regulating Xin, Yi and Li
    using Xin to lead Qi, 1, 2, 91
    Xin must be calm/quiet, 53
    Xin raises up the Fighting Spirit, 71
    Xin raises up the Spirit of Vitality, 92
Yang, Lu-Shan, v, vii
Yang style Taijiquan, v, vii, xi
Yi,
    see also Broken Jin, under Jin
    see also Regulating Xin, Yi and Li
    coordinating Yi and Qi, viii, 2, 95
    keeping the Yi on your Dan Tian, 58
    manifesting the Yi on the palms, 82
    the opponent's Yi, 46
    the Yi keeps the Xin under control, 71, 92
    Yi and Qi are the master (sovereign), 94, 95
    Yi and Qi arrive, Jin follows, 91
    Yi controls body, viii
    Yi generates Jin, 65, 82
    Yi leads Qi, 1,2, 40, 55, 65, 70-72, 82, 91
Yi Jing, 44
Yield, 15, 21, 26, 63, 65, 66, 81, 82, 85, 99
Yin and Yang, 23, 24, 36, 42, 44, 58, 59, 63-67,
    69-71, 92, 94, 98, 101, 103
Yin Primary Qi Channels, 92
Yin Yang Symbol/Circle, 97, 98, 99
Yin, 26, 59
Yintang Palace (M-HN-3), see Third Eye
Yongquan cavity (K-1), 91, 92
Yu Huan Xue (residence of Spiritual Fetus), 69
Zhong Gong (Central Palace or Central
    Equilibrium), 79, 86
Zhou (Elbow), 31, 35, 78, 79, 84, 85, 87, 88, 89

BOOKS FROM YMAA

ANALYSIS OF GENUINE KARATE 1 & 2
ANALYSIS OF SHAOLIN CHIN NA 2ND ED
ART AND SCIENCE OF STAFF FIGHTING
THE ART AND SCIENCE OF SELF-DEFENSE
ART AND SCIENCE OF STICK FIGHTING
ART OF HOJO UNDO
BAGUAZHANG
CHINESE TUI NA MASSAGE
COMPREHENSIVE APPLICATIONS OF SHAOLIN CHIN NA
DAO DE JING: A QIGONG INTERPRETATION
ESSENCE OF SHAOLIN WHITE CRANE
FIGHT LIKE A PHYSICIST
JUDO ADVANTAGE
JUJI GATAME ENCYCLOPEDIA
KRAV MAGA COMBATIVES
KRAV MAGA FUNDAMENTAL STRATEGIES
KRAV MAGA PROFESSIONAL TACTICS
KRAV MAGA WEAPON DEFENSES
LITTLE BLACK BOOK OF VIOLENCE
LIUHEBAFA FIVE CHARACTER SECRETS
MARTIAL ARTS OF VIETNAM
MEDITATIONS ON VIOLENCE
MERIDIAN QIGONG EXERCISES
NORTHERN SHAOLIN SWORD
PRINCIPLES OF TRADITIONAL CHINESE MEDICINE
QIGONG FOR HEALTH & MARTIAL ARTS
QIGONG FOR TREATING COMMON AILMENTS
QIGONG MASSAGE
QIGONG MEDITATION: EMBRYONIC BREATHING
QIGONG GRAND CIRCULATION
QIGONG MEDITATION: SMALL CIRCULATION
QIGONG, THE SECRET OF YOUTH: DA MO'S CLASSICS
ROOT OF CHINESE QIGONG
SAMBO ENCYCLOPEDIA
SIMPLE QIGONG EXERCISES FOR HEALTH, 3RD ED.
SIMPLIFIED TAI CHI CHUAN, 2ND ED.
SPOTTING DANGER BEFORE IT SPOTS YOU
SPOTTING DANGER BEFORE IT SPOTS YOUR KIDS
SPOTTING DANGER BEFORE IT SPOTS YOUR TEENS
SPOTTING DANGER FOR TRAVELERS
SUMO FOR MIXED MARTIAL ARTS
SURVIVING ARMED ASSAULTS
TAI CHI BALL QIGONG
TAI CHI CHIN NA
TAI CHI CHUAN CLASSICAL YANG STYLE
TAI CHI CHUAN MARTIAL APPLICATIONS
TAI CHI CHUAN MARTIAL POWER
TAI CHI CONCEPTS AND EXPERIMENTS
TAI CHI IN 10 WEEKS
TAI CHI PUSH HANDS
TAI CHI QIGONG TAI CHI SECRETS OF THE WU & LI STYLES
TAI CHI SECRETS OF THE WU STYLE
TAI CHI SECRETS OF THE YANG STYLE
TAI CHI SWORD: CLASSICAL YANG STYLE
TAI CHI CHUAN THEORY OF DR. YANG, JWING-MING
TRADITIONAL CHINESE HEALTH SECRETS
TRUE WELLNESS SERIES (MIND, HEART, GUT)
WING CHUN IN-DEPTH
XINGYIQUAN

AND MANY MORE . . .

VIDEOS FROM YMAA

ANALYSIS OF SHAOLIN CHIN NA
ART AND SCIENCE OF SELF DEFENSE
ART AND SCIENCE OF STAFF FIGHTING
ART AND SCIENCE STICK FIGHTING
BAGUA FOR BEGINNERS 1 & 2
BEGINNER TAI CHI FOR HEALTH
CHEN TAI CHI FOR BEGINNERS
CHIN NA IN-DEPTH SERIES
INTRODUCTION TO QI GONG FOR BEGINNERS
JOINT LOCKS
KUNG FU BODY CONDITIONING 1 & 2
KUNG FU FOR KIDS AND TEENS SERIES
MERIDIAN QIGONG
NORTHERN SHAOLIN SWORD
QI GONG 30-DAY CHALLENGE
QI GONG FOR HEALTHY JOINTS
QIGONG FOR WOMEN WITH DAISY LEE
QIGONG GRAND CIRCULATION
QIGONG MASSAGE
QIGONG: 15 MINUTES TO HEALTH
SANCHIN KATA: TRADITIONAL TRAINING FOR KARATE POWER
SHAOLIN KUNG FU FUNDAMENTAL TRAINING: COURSES 1 & 2
SHAOLIN LONG FIST KUNG FU BEGINNER—INTERMEDIATE—ADVANCED
SHAOLIN SABER: BASIC SEQUENCES
SHAOLIN STAFF: BASIC SEQUENCES
SHAOLIN WHITE CRANE GONG FU BASIC TRAINING SERIES
SIMPLE QIGONG EXERCISES FOR HEALTH
SIMPLE QIGONG EXERCISES FOR ARTHRITIS RELIEF
SIMPLE QIGONG EXERCISES FOR BACK PAIN RELIEF
SIMPLIFIED TAI CHI CHUAN: 24 & 48 POSTURES
SPOTTING DANGER SERIES
SWORD: FUNDAMENTAL TRAINING
TAI CHI BALL QIGONG SERIES
TAI CHI BALL WORKOUT FOR BEGINNERS
TAI CHI CHUAN CLASSICAL YANG STYLE
TAI CHI FIGHTING SET
TAI CHI FIT: 24 FORM
TAI CHI FIT: FOR WOMEN
TAI CHI FIT: OVER 50
TAI CHI FIT OVER 50: BALANCE EXERCISES
TAI CHI FIT OVER 50: SEATED WORKOUT
TAI CHI FIT OVER 60: GENTLE EXERCISES
TAI CHI FIT OVER 60: HEALTHY JOINTS
TAI CHI FOR WOMEN
TAI CHI QIGONG
TAI CHI PRINCIPLES FOR HEALTHY AGING
TAI CHI PUSHING HANDS SERIES
TAI CHI SWORD: CLASSICAL YANG STYLE
TAI CHI SWORD FOR BEGINNERS
TAIJI & SHAOLIN STAFF: FUNDAMENTAL TRAINING
TAIJI CHIN NA IN-DEPTH
TAIJI SABER CLASSICAL YANG STYLE
TAIJI WRESTLING
UNDERSTANDING QIGONG SERIES
WHITE CRANE HARD & SOFT QIGONG
YANG TAI CHI FOR BEGINNERS
YOQI QIGONG FLOW FOR STRESS RELIEF
WU TAI CHI FOR BEGINNERS
WUDANG KUNG FU: FUNDAMENTAL TRAINING
WUDANG SWORD
WUDANG TAIJIQUAN
XINGYIQUAN
YANG TAI CHI FOR BEGINNERS

AND MANY MORE . . .

more products available from . . .

YMAA Publication Center, Inc. 楊氏東方文化出版中心

1-800-669-8892 • info@ymaa.com • www.ymaa.com

Printed in the USA
CPSIA information can be obtained
at www.ICGtesting.com
JSHW070853140224
R13335300001B/R133353PG56550JSX00001B/1